Contents

NHSAcronym – the handy app at your fingertips
Download the NHSAcronym app to your iPhone or iPad
so that you have the definition of over 600 commonly
used acronyms in the NHS at your fingertips.

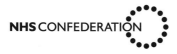
NHSCONFEDERATION

The NHS Confederation is the membership body that brings together the full range of organisations that commission and provide NHS services.

We work with our members and health and social care partners to help the NHS guarantee high standards of care for patients and the public by:
- influencing health policy and representing members' views to Government, Parliament, policymakers and the public
- making sense of the whole health system with our publications and information services
- championing good practice at events, in workshops and forums, and through partnerships
- supporting the health industry with the help of the NHS Employers organisation and our offices in Brussels, Wales and Northern Ireland.

We work with our networks and forums to bring together the views and perspectives of different parts of the healthcare system and support our members on issues of specific concern.

BME Leadership Forum • Community Health Services Forum • Hospitals Forum • Mental Health Network • NHS Partners Network • Urgent and Emergency Care Forum • working with NHS Clinical Commissioners

We also offer the opportunity for organisations working across the wider health and social care industry to be a part of the NHS Confederation as associate partners.

Further information
To find out more about the NHS Confederation, please visit our website at **www.nhsconfed.org**

Sponsor's foreword

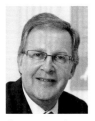

2013 is the year in which the NHS spun on its axis. As it reaches its 65th birthday, we find ourselves in a radical new environment where clinical commissioning groups, led by clinicians in primary care, are responsible for shaping a health service fit for the future, one that meets the changing needs and expectations of patients and taxpayers. This vision inspires many opportunities but, as the report by Robert Francis QC into the care failings at Mid Staffs shows, a service as all-encompassing as the NHS can never afford to be complacent.

NHS staff, especially nurses, have never before been under such scrutiny, but the reality is that mistakes happen when competent people are over-stretched. It is our responsibility to work closely with trusts to ensure that the tens of thousands of temporary workers we manage on behalf of the NHS are properly trained, rigorously vetted and ascribe to the values and behaviours covered by the six Cs: care, compassion, competence, communication, courage and commitment.

As an active participant to changes in the NHS, NHS Professionals will be engaging in a debate with procurement teams and framework providers to develop their understanding of the tangible benefits of procuring a stable supply of temporary staff under a managed services agreement. We want to drive consideration of broader objectives than simply hourly rates and agency commission charges, such as compliance with NHS Employment Check standards; management information that helps trusts address the underlying demand for bank and locum work; and appropriate fill strategies.

We are delighted to be supporting *The NHS handbook* again – a vital resource that aims to reflect the views, perspectives and opinions across our unrivalled healthcare system.

Stephen Dangerfield
Chief Executive
NHS Professionals

www.nhsp.co.uk
NHS Professionals
NHS Professionals
@nhsworkforce

Foreword

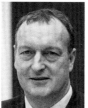

April 2013 saw the dawn of a new NHS in England. Major changes to the health service have altered the NHS landscape, introducing a new structure, new organisations and bodies, and new remits and responsibilities, which provide big opportunities to improve healthcare.

The concise NHS handbook 2013/14 is the essential guide to the new system, helping you to make sense of and navigate the post-April 2013 NHS. This succinct edition sets out the structure of the health service in England, details the new commissioning landscape and breaks down how healthcare is provided.

Lessons from Mid Staffordshire and the Francis Report have renewed the NHS's focus on quality, and our updated *Quality and safety* and *Accountability and regulation* chapters provide a detailed overview of the mechanisms and structures in place to ensure the highest quality care for patients.

The concise NHS handbook 2013/14 is supported by advertising from a number of organisations we work alongside, and I am particularly grateful to NHS Professionals for kindly agreeing to support this year's edition.

I hope you will find this timely guide invaluable in 2013/14, whether you are new to the health sector or have a wealth of experience. At the NHS Confederation, we will continue our work to join up the views, perspectives and opinions of each and every part of the healthcare system over the coming year.

If you have any comments or suggestions for future editions of the handbook, please contact our publications team on 020 7799 6666 or email **publishingteam@nhsconfed.org**

Mike Farrar CBE
Chief Executive
NHS Confederation

Introduction

On a typical day, the National Health Service in England interacts with over a million patients:
- 836,000 people visit their GP practice or practice nurse
- 389,000 people have contact with community health services
- 60,000 people visit accident and emergency departments
- 192,000 attend outpatient departments
- 114,000 people are in hospital after being admitted as an emergency
- 44,000 people are in hospital for planned treatment
- 108,500 patients receive dental treatment
- 13,000 emergency patient journeys by ambulance take place
- 2.6 million prescription items are dispensed.

This year the NHS marks its 65th anniversary, but its underlying values remain the same as when it was founded. These originate from the 1944 white paper, *A national health service*, which stated that:

> The Government want to ensure that in future every man, woman and child can rely on getting all the advice and treatment and care they may need in matters of personal health; that what they shall get shall be the best medical and other facilities available; that their getting these shall not depend on whether they can pay for them or any other factor irrelevant to the real need.

Both society and the health service have altered almost beyond recognition since then: the NHS has had to move with the times to take advantage of scientific and technological advances, as well as political, social and economic change. Major reform programmes have been under way for more than a decade – the latest implemented in April 2013. But the NHS still strives to provide a broadly comprehensive service, mostly free to all at the point of need. As the NHS Constitution, devised in 2008 for the health service in England, expresses it: 'Everyone counts. We maximise our resources for the benefit of the whole community, and make sure nobody is excluded, discriminated against or left behind.'

The NHS is based on common principles throughout the four constituent parts of the United Kingdom, although its structure in each is quite distinctive – and increasingly so. It has always adapted its shape to the particular administrative and geographical conditions of England, Scotland, Wales and Northern Ireland. But since devolution in 1999, the divergence in structure has become more marked (see pages 133–135). The NHS has also pursued different priorities in each of the four countries.

The Scottish Parliament, the Welsh Assembly and the Northern Ireland Assembly are responsible for oversight of the NHS in their parts of the UK, and the Scottish Government Health Directorates, the Welsh Department for Health and Social Services and Northern Ireland's Department of Health, Social Services and Public Safety provide strategic leadership. Health services in the Isle of Man and the Channel Islands are not part of the NHS.

As policy and legislation from the European Union began to have an increasing impact on the UK health service, the NHS European Office was set up. Established in 2007 and based in Brussels and London, it is part of the NHS Confederation. Its work includes:

- monitoring EU developments that have an impact on the NHS
- informing NHS organisations of EU affairs
- promoting the priorities and interests of the NHS to European institutions
- advising NHS organisations of EU funding opportunities.

www.nhsconfed.org/europe

01 The structure of the NHS in England

Ultimate responsibility for the NHS lies with Parliament. At a strategic level, with the implementation of the Government's NHS reorganisation in April 2013, the Department of Health passed much of its day-to-day responsibility to NHS England and other arm's-length bodies. At an operational level, clinical commissioning groups occupy a pivotal position, while foundation trusts, NHS trusts and independent healthcare organisations and contractors provide the services.

Parliament

As the NHS is financed mainly through taxation it relies on Parliament for funds, and must account to it for their use. Parliament scrutinises the service through debates, MPs' questions to ministers and select committees. These procedures mean that the Government has to publicly explain and defend its policies for the NHS in England.

Role of the Secretary of State and health ministers

Currently five ministers, all appointed by the Prime Minister to the Department of Health, are responsible in Parliament for health and social care. Although the details of their portfolios change periodically, they provide the DH with political leadership and are responsible for deciding strategy and policy, and for agreeing overall resource levels with the Chancellor and the Prime Minister, as well as priorities for distributing resources, based on the strategy and policy framework.

The DH's ministers comprise the Secretary of State and currently a minister of state responsible for care and support, as well as three parliamentary under-secretaries of state: one responsible for health, one for public health and the other, who sits in the House of Lords, for quality.

The Secretary of State is a member of the cabinet and has overall responsibility for strategic leadership of the NHS and social care system. The Secretary of State retains an overarching duty to *promote* a comprehensive health service – a founding principle of the NHS – but ministers are not responsible for *providing* or commissioning services directly, passing this duty to new bodies such as NHS England by way of a 'mandate' (see page 18). The Government believes that previous statutory arrangements encouraged ministers to 'micromanage' parts of the NHS. The Secretary of State must produce an annual report for Parliament setting out how the NHS has performed in the previous year.

The new NHS structure

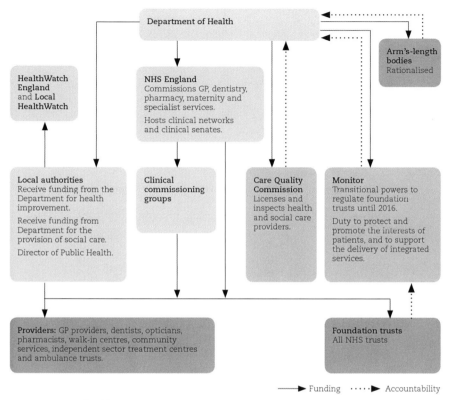

Department of Health

Arm's-length bodies
Rationalised

HealthWatch England and Local HealthWatch

NHS England
Commissions GP, dentistry, pharmacy, maternity and specialist services.

Hosts clinical networks and clinical senates.

Local authorities
Receive funding from the Department for health improvement.

Receive funding from Department for the provision of social care.

Director of Public Health.

Clinical commissioning groups

Care Quality Commission
Licenses and inspects health and social care providers.

Monitor
Transitional powers to regulate foundation trusts until 2016.

Duty to protect and promote the interests of patients, and to support the delivery of integrated services.

Providers: GP providers, dentists, opticians, pharmacists, walk-in centres, community services, independent sector treatment centres and ambulance trusts.

Foundation trusts
All NHS trusts

⟶ Funding ·····▶ Accountability

Source: Department of Health

Further information
The National Health Service and Public Health Service in England: Secretary of State's annual report 2011/2012, HM Government, July 2012.

Select committees
Select committees consider policy issues, scrutinise the Government's work and spending, and examine proposals for legislation. Members are drawn from backbench MPs of all parties. Four select committees, each comprising backbench MPs representing the major parties, are particularly relevant to the NHS. They are all able to summon ministers, civil servants and NHS employees to give oral or written evidence to their inquiries, usually in public. Their reports are published throughout the parliamentary session.

Health committee

The health committee's role is 'to examine the expenditure, administration and policy of the Department of Health and its associated bodies'. The committee now also exercises on Parliament's behalf the power to hold the General Medical Council (see page 105) to account, and has extended this to include the Nursing and Midwifery Council (see page 105). It also holds regular annual review meetings with the Care Quality Commission (see page 99) and Monitor (see page 100). The committee has a maximum of 11 members.

www.parliament.uk

Public accounts committee

The public accounts committee scrutinises all public spending and is concerned with ensuring the NHS is operating with economy, efficiency and effectiveness. Its inquiries are based on reports about the service's 'value for money', produced by the Comptroller and Auditor General, who heads the National Audit Office (see page 103). It aims to draw lessons from past successes and failures that can be applied to future activity. The committee has 16 members, and is traditionally chaired by an Opposition MP.

www.parliament.uk

www.nao.gov.uk

Communities and local government committee

The communities and local government committee monitors the policy, administration and spending of the Department of Communities and Local Government, and so has an interest in councils' public health responsibilities and in health and wellbeing boards (see page 19). One of its recent reports examined local authorities' role in health issues. It has 11 members.

www.parliament.uk

Public administration committee

The public administration committee examines reports from the Parliamentary and Health Service Ombudsman (see page 97). Its remit now includes responsibility for scrutinising third sector policy. It has 11 members.

www.parliament.uk

www.ombudsman.org.uk

Department of Health

The Government has fundamentally changed the DH's role. It is no longer the headquarters of the NHS nor directly manages any NHS organisations. Its main responsibilities include:

- setting national policy on health and adult social care and maintaining legislation
- setting strategy and outcomes for health and adult social care
- providing leadership
- managing relationships throughout the health and care system
- securing resources and accounting for them
- speaking for the UK on international health issues.

The DH has strategic responsibility for a range of arm's-length bodies, including:

- NHS England (see page 16)
- Monitor (see page 100)
- Care Quality Commission (see page 99)
- Public Health England (see page 38)
- Health Education England (see page 124)
- NHS Trust Development Authority (see page 22).

Although the DH is not responsible for the NHS in Scotland, Wales and Northern Ireland, it has UK-wide responsibility for international and European Union business and for:

- coordinating plans to cope with a flu pandemic
- licensing and safety of medicines and medical devices
- ethical issues such as abortion and embryology.

Managing the DH

The DH comprises five directorates:

- NHS
- adult social care
- public health
- partnerships and engagement
- operations.

Its two most senior staff, of equal rank, are the permanent secretary and the chief medical officer. These posts are not political appointments and do not change with a change of government. The permanent secretary is responsible for running the department day to day and is its chief accounting officer. The DH's chief medical officer is the UK Government's principal medical adviser and the professional head of all medical staff in England.

Other DH chief professional officers, who provide expert knowledge in specialist health and social care disciplines to ministers, other government departments and the Prime Minister, are:
• director of nursing
• chief dental officer
• chief health professions officer
• chief pharmaceutical officer
• chief scientific officer.

Further information
Department of Health accounting officer system statement, DH, August 2012.
Department of Health annual report and accounts 2011–12, TSO, October 2012.
www.dh.gov.uk

Arm's-length bodies

An arm's-length body (ALB) is an organisation working at national level, but at 'arm's length' from the DH. They have existed since the NHS was set up in 1948. As standalone organisations, ALBs work closely with the local NHS, social care services and other ALBs to carry out specific functions. They vary in size but normally have boards, employ staff and publish accounts. They are accountable to the DH and sometimes directly to Parliament. Most receive substantial funding from the DH.

They include special health authorities, executive agencies and non-departmental public bodies, which are set up when ministers want independent advice without direct influence from Whitehall departments.

Their roles are:
• regulating the health and social care system and workforce
• establishing national standards and protecting patients and public
• providing central services to the NHS.

NHS England

NHS England, originally known as the NHS Commissioning Board, is a pivotal part of the new structure. It provides leadership for commissioning (see page 29) and will be nationally accountable for the outcomes the NHS achieves. NHS England has overall responsibility for a budget in 2013/14 of £95 billion, of which it will allocate £65 billion directly to clinical commissioning groups (see page 19).

The 2010 white paper, *Liberating the NHS*, promised that NHS England would be 'a lean and expert organisation, free from day-to-day political interference, with a commissioning model that draws from best international practice', adding that: 'It will not manage providers or be the NHS headquarters'.

NHS England and its key relationships

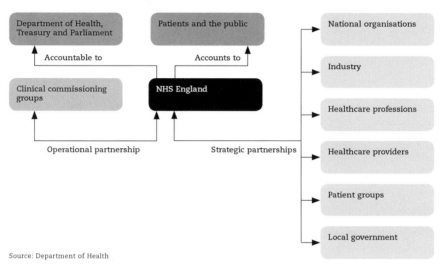

Source: Department of Health

Its main functions include:
- overseeing a comprehensive system of clinical commissioning groups (CCGs) responsible for commissioning most healthcare services
- commissioning directly services that CCGs cannot commission, such as primary care and specialised services (see page 29)
- overseeing the commissioning budget and ensuring value for money
- developing commissioning guidance, standard contracts, pricing mechanisms and information standards
- agreeing and achieving improved outcomes
- improving quality by promoting consistent national standards
- promoting innovative ways to integrate care
- reducing inequalities and promoting equality and diversity
- engaging public, patients and carers, championing their interests and ensuring wider access to information
- fostering choice, and with Monitor developing guidance on how choice and competition can be applied to particular services
- overseeing emergency planning
- with its partners, developing a medium-term strategy for the NHS.

As well as a chair and six non-executive directors, NHS England's senior team comprises:
• chief executive
• medical director
• chief nursing officer
• chief operating officer and deputy chief executive
• national director – policy
• national director – commissioning development
• chief financial officer
• national director – human resources
• national director – patients and information
• four regional directors.

It has more than 6,000 staff, two-thirds deployed locally managing relationships with CCGs and performing direct commissioning in 27 local area teams. In addition, regional sectors cover London, the South, the North, and Midlands and East. Its annual running costs are £527 million.
www.england.nhs.uk

The Mandate
The Secretary of State sets NHS England a formal mandate specifying all the Government's requirements and expectations for the NHS for the next two years. For 2013/14 it is structured around five key areas:
• preventing people dying prematurely
• enhancing quality of life for people with long-term conditions
• helping people recover from ill health or injury
• ensuring people have a positive experience of care
• treating and caring for people in a safe environment, and protecting them from avoidable harm.

NHS England must produce an annual business plan detailing how it intends to achieve the mandate's objectives (see page 30), and report on its performance at the end of the year. As an independent arm's-length body, NHS England is also directly accountable to Parliament.

Further information
The Mandate: a mandate from the Government to the NHS Commissioning Board: April 2013 to March 2015, DH, November 2012.
http://mandate.dh.gov.uk

Clinical commissioning groups

The 211 clinical commissioning groups are independent statutory bodies, formed from the GP practices in their area: all 8,000-plus GP practices in England are members of a CCG.

Covering populations from 68,000 to over 900,000, CCGs are collectively responsible for £65 billion of the £95 billion NHS commissioning budget. They commission services across a range of clinical areas (see page 31), including hospital services, emergency and urgent care, ambulance services, community services and mental healthcare, but do not commission primary care nor national or regional specialised services, which are part of NHS England's remit.

Each CCG's governing body is free to decide organisational form and management strategy, taking account of guidance and legislation. However, they are required to meet in public and publish minutes, as well as details of contracts with health services. They must not spend more than £25 per head of population per year on running costs.

Further information
The functions of clinical commissioning groups (updated to reflect the final Health and Social Care Act 2012), DH, June 2012.

NHS Commissioning Assembly
The NHS Commissioning Assembly is designed to create shared leadership nationally and locally between NHS England and CCGs. It is intended to enable them to co-produce national strategy and direction, embed principles for working together and create a common voice, connecting leaders within the NHS commissioning system and beyond.

Health and wellbeing boards

Each of the 152 upper-tier and unitary local authorities has a health and wellbeing board (HWB) to act as a forum for local commissioners across the NHS, social care, public health and other services. HWBs aim to develop a shared understanding of local need, develop joint local priorities and encourage commissioners to work in a more integrated, 'joined-up' manner.

NHS Clinical Commissioners is the only independent membership
organisation exclusively for clinical commissioning groups. Its purpose is
to help CCGs achieve the best healthcare and health outcomes for their
communities and patients. It is designed to give CCGs an influential voice
from the front line to the wider NHS, national bodies, Government,
Parliament and the media, drawing on the experience of its three founding
partners – the NHS Alliance, the National Association of Primary Care and
the NHS Confederation.
www.nhscc.org

The main functions of HWBs are:
• assessing the local population's needs and leading the joint strategic
  needs assessment and joint health and wellbeing strategy (see page 34)
• promoting integration and partnership across an area – for example, by
  promoting joined-up commissioning plans across the NHS, social care
  and public health
• supporting integration of care
• scrutinising major service redesign.

HWBs are intended to give local authorities influence over NHS
commissioning, and corresponding influence for NHS commissioners on
public health and social care. They have a statutory duty to involve users
and the public. The Government hopes that by involving democratically
elected representatives and patient representatives it will strengthen the
democratic legitimacy of commissioning decisions, as well as provide a
forum for challenge, discussion and involving local people.

Membership of HWBs includes:
• at least one councillor
• director of adult social services
• director of children's services
• director of public health
• local HealthWatch representative (see page 94)
• a representative of each local CCG
• others the local authority or HWB may choose.

Local authorities decide for themselves the number of councillors on an
HWB, and can insist they are a majority. HWBs decide for themselves how
to involve local providers.

NHS England must take the HWB's views into account in its annual assessment of a CCG, and consult it on the CCG's contribution to achieving the joint health and wellbeing strategy (see page 35).

Further information
Stronger together: how health and wellbeing boards can work effectively with local providers, NHS Confederation and partners, January 2013.
Liberating the NHS: increasing democratic legitimacy in health, DH, July 2010.

Clinical senates and strategic clinical networks

The 12 clinical senates provide strategic clinical advice and leadership across a broad geographical area to CCGs, health and wellbeing boards and NHS England. They are not focused on a particular condition but, for example, may help identify aspects of healthcare with potential to improve outcomes and value, or help convince the public of the need for service changes by providing clinical leadership and credibility.

Clinical senates should not constrain a CCG's activities or be involved in assessing commissioners' performance. They cannot veto proposals but recommend where further thinking is needed. Senates are non-statutory advisory bodies with no executive authority or legal obligations, so must work collaboratively with commissioning organisations.

Membership is decided locally but must be multi-professional and span a variety of commissioning and provider organisations. A core steering group of members form the senate council, while the senate assembly provides access to a broad range of experts.

Clinical senates are intended to have a particularly close relationship with strategic clinical networks. NHS England has set up and supported these to advise commissioners, support change projects and improve outcomes. They are designed to help clinicians gather and share insights into complex conditions for which treatment is often delivered across different settings. They cover:
• cancer
• cardiovascular disease
• maternity and children
• mental health, dementia and neurological conditions.

They will be established for up to five years, depending on the amount of change needed in a specific area.

Foundation trusts

Foundation trusts run hospitals, specialist care centres, mental healthcare, community health and ambulance services. First established in 2004, they are independent public benefit organisations, modelled on cooperatives and mutual societies, but remain part of the NHS. They are still accountable to Parliament, but local people have a say in running them by becoming members or governors (see page 90). Monitor, the independent regulator of foundation trusts (see page 100), has powers to intervene in how a trust is run if it fails to meet standards or breaches its terms of authorisation. The Care Quality Commission (see page 99) is responsible for inspecting the performance of foundation trusts, as it is for all other NHS organisations.

Foundation status bestows more freedom on organisations than they had as NHS trusts. This includes:
• the ability to retain any operating surpluses – for example, from land sales – and access to capital from both the public and private sectors; the amount a foundation trust can borrow is determined by a formula based on its ability to repay the loan, and governed by the prudential borrowing code set by Monitor
• a new power to earn up to 49 per cent of their income from treating private patients, though foundation trusts must publish separate accounts for NHS and private-funded services
• an obligation to achieve national standards like the rest of the NHS, but freedom to decide how they do this
• powers to establish private companies
• the ability to vary staff pay from nationally agreed terms and conditions.

By 2013 there were 145 foundation trusts, including 41 mental health trusts and five ambulance trusts. About 100 NHS trusts remain, of which about half are expected to progress to foundation status, according to the NHS Trust Development Authority. The remainder face mergers or other solutions.

NHS Trust Development Authority
The NTDA is responsible for guiding NHS trusts seeking foundation status. As well as managing the 'FT pipeline', this includes managing performance and intervening in poorly performing trusts.

Further information
Toward high quality, sustainable services: planning guidance for NHS trust boards for 2013/14, NHS Trust Development Authority, April 2013.
Building the NHS Trust Development Authority, NHS, January 2012.
www.ntda.nhs.uk

Spotlight on policy **academic health science networks**
The 15 academic health science networks (AHSNs) are designed to improve the identification, adoption and spread of innovation in the NHS. Their aim is to 'align education, clinical research, informatics, training and education and healthcare delivery'. They cover all of England, each with a population of 3–5 million, though they are configured in different ways. Effective cross-sector governance and partnership working will be key to their success.

Further information
Briefing 246: Academic health science networks: engaging with innovation and improvement, NHS Confederation, June 2012.

Independent providers

By using independent providers – private sector companies, voluntary organisations and social enterprises – to offer care to NHS patients, the health service has been able to expand capacity and improve choice. The previous Government introduced this policy in 2002 – believing that competition would prompt the NHS to improve its response to patients' needs – and extended it in 2008. The current Government has extended it further.

Now 'any qualified provider' (AQP) may offer services to NHS patients, though the areas of care that are a priority for implementing AQP are decided locally. The Government expects the policy will improve quality and access, help tackle inequalities and encourage innovation.

To qualify, providers must:
• be registered with the CQC and be licensed by Monitor (see page 102) or meet equivalent assurance requirements
• meet the terms and conditions of the NHS standard contract (see page 33), which involves abiding by the NHS Constitution (see page 93), relevant guidance and law

- accept NHS prices
- guarantee to meet agreed service requirements and comply with referral protocols.

In 2011/12 the independent sector provided more than 345,000 procedures for NHS elective patients, an 11 per cent increase on 2010/11.

Further information
Operational guidance to the NHS: extending patient choice of provider, DH, July 2011.
AQP Resource Centre **www.supply2health.nhs.uk**

The private sector
Traditionally, private healthcare providers in the UK tended to concentrate on secondary care, but new entrants to the market in the past decade have looked for opportunities in primary and community care too. They have also become major suppliers of diagnostic services to the NHS.

The previous Government initially encouraged private sector companies to set up treatment centres (see page 59) to carry out elective surgery and diagnostic tests for NHS patients under five-year contracts to help alleviate waiting times: by 2011/12 these centres accounted for about 40 per cent of NHS-funded procedures undertaken outside the NHS. They paved the way for private companies gradually to play a bigger role, and volumes of services they provide to the NHS rose rapidly.

The third sector
The 'third sector' comprises the range of institutions that fall between the public and private sectors, and includes small local community and voluntary groups, large and small registered charities, foundations, trusts, cooperatives and social enterprises. They often provide inpatient and outpatient mental health services, sexual health services, drug rehabilitation and palliative care. Many smaller voluntary organisations play a crucial part in community services, particularly for vulnerable and excluded groups, and are often able to bridge divides between statutory services. The aim is that they should become 'equal players' in providing services.

About 35,000 such organisations provide health or social care. Total funding for these services amounts to £12 billion a year, with just over half from the public sector – 36 per cent of which is for healthcare and 62 per cent for social care.

NHS Partners Network

NHS Partners Network (NHSPN) is the trade association representing a wide range of independent sector providers of NHS services in acute, diagnostic, primary and community care, as well as dental services. The NHSPN was incorporated into the NHS Confederation in 2007. Its members are drawn from both the 'for profit' and 'not for profit' sectors, including large international hospital groups and small, specialist providers. Members are committed to working in partnership with the NHS and to the values in the NHS Constitution.
www.nhsconfed.org/nhspn

A health and care voluntary sector strategic partner programme has been launched by the DH, NHS England and Public Health England (see page 38) to invest in a number of national voluntary organisations and help improve communication with the sector. It builds on a previous scheme that had 18 members, through which the DH estimated it reached 300,000 organisations across the sector.

Social enterprises

Social enterprises are organisations run on business lines, but which reinvest profits in the community or in service developments. They take different forms, and may include cooperatives, trusts or community interest companies. They number 68,000, contribute £24 billion to the economy and employ 800,000 people. An estimated 6,000 social enterprises deliver health and social care within the NHS. They involve patients and staff in designing and delivering services, improving quality and tailoring services to meet patients' needs.

In 2008 NHS staff were given a 'right to request' to set up a social enterprise to offer services previously provided in-house. Building on the 'right to request', the current Government has launched its own 'right to provide' scheme and extended it to all health and social care staff. By 2012, 57 social enterprises involving 25,000 staff had been 'spun out' from the NHS.

Further information
Office for Civil Society www.civilsociety.co.uk
Social Enterprise Coalition www.socialenterprise.org.uk

Independent contractors

Most GPs, dentists, opticians and pharmacists are independent contractors. They are not employed directly by the NHS but are contracted to provide services to patients for which they are paid by the NHS. Independent contractors may also carry out private work not funded by the NHS. Therefore within an individual practice, such as a GP or dental practice, the staff are employed directly by the contract holder and not the NHS.

02 Commissioning

Commissioning is the process by which the NHS decides what services are needed, acquires them and then ensures they are being provided appropriately. It involves assessing the population's needs and deciding which are priorities, procuring the services to meet them and managing the providers.

The origins of commissioning can be traced to the advent of the internal market in 1991 and the division of the NHS into purchasers and providers. Then it was referred to as 'purchasing'.

The Government has argued that 'commissioning has been too remote from the patients it is intended to serve', and decided responsibility for it should rest with healthcare professionals rather than managerial organisations. Healthcare professionals especially play a critical role in influencing NHS expenditure – for example, through referral and prescribing decisions. Clinical commissioning therefore gives them financial accountability for the consequences of their decisions. Clinical commissioning groups (see page 19), NHS England (see page 16) and local authorities are now the main commissioners of healthcare.

Further information
Liberating the NHS: commissioning for patients, DH, July 2010.

The basics
The commissioning process comprises three broad activities – strategic planning, procurement and management – and is based on an eight-step cycle:

Assessing needs – systematically understanding the local population's health and care needs

Describing services and gap analysis – reviewing current services and defining the gaps (or over-provision) based on needs

Deciding priorities – using evidence of cost-effectiveness and based on a defensible ethical framework, deciding what to commission with available funds

Risk management – understanding key health and healthcare risks and deciding on a strategy to manage them

Strategic options – combining information into a single strategic commissioning plan that outlines how objectives will be met

Contract implementation – implementing the strategic plan through contracting

Provider development – including care pathway redesign and demand management, helping providers to improve – or decommission – services or introducing new providers

Managing provider performance – monitoring against contracts, using key performance indicators.

In addition, sound commissioning attempts to shift towards services that are personal, sensitive to individual need, and which maintain independence and dignity. It must focus on services and interventions that will achieve better health, promote inclusion and tackle health inequalities. It must also try to reorient towards promoting health and wellbeing, investing to reduce the future costs of ill health. It has therefore outgrown its fairly narrow traditional base of needs assessment and contracting.

NHS England's role

NHS England directly commissions some services. These include:

- primary medical, dental, pharmacy and optical services, and other dental services
- specialised services
- some specific public health screening and immunisation services
- prison healthcare
- military healthcare.

NHS England spends £12.6 billion annually on commissioning primary care: obvious conflicts of interest prevent CCGs commissioning most primary care, but they are expected to help NHS England improve the quality of these services, and it can ask CCGs to carry out some commissioning functions relating to primary care on its behalf. CCGs are also expected to influence how NHS England commissions other services.

In addition, NHS England directly commissions specialised services – those with low patient numbers but which need a critical mass of patients to make treatment centres cost-effective. They are provided in relatively few specialist centres to catchment populations of more than 1 million people. As they are high-cost, low-volume treatments, the risk to an individual or group of CCGs of having to fund expensive, unpredictable activity would be prohibitive. Specialised services account for £11.8 billion a year, about 10 per cent of the NHS budget. NHS England's role is to plan, specify and procure, deliver and improve specialised services.

Putting patients first

Putting patients first is NHS England's three-year business plan, covering 2013/14 to 2015/16. The plan includes an 11-point scorecard, which NHS England will introduce for measuring performance on key priorities. Following the Francis Report (see page 82) these priorities include feedback from patients, their families and NHS staff.

The 11 key priorities on the scorecard are:
- satisfied patients
- motivated, positive NHS staff
- preventing people from dying prematurely
- enhancing quality of life for people with long-term conditions
- helping people to recover from episodes of ill health or following injury
- ensuring people have a positive experience of care
- treating and caring for people in a safe environment; and protecting them from avoidable harm
- promoting equality and reducing inequalities in health outcomes
- adhering to NHS Constitution rights and pledges
- becoming an excellent organisation
- high-quality financial management.

The business plan outlines eight key areas that NHS England will use to achieve the 11 priorities: supporting, ensuring and developing the commissioning system; direct commissioning; emergency preparedness; partnership for quality; strategy, research and innovation for outcomes and growth; clinical and professional leadership; world-class customer service; and developing commissioning support.

Further information
Putting patients first: the NHS England business plan 2013/14–2015/16, NHS England, April 2013.

In addition, NHS England provides national leadership for commissioning. For example, it sets commissioning guidelines on the basis of clinically approved quality standards developed with advice from NICE (see page 101), and designs model NHS contracts for CCGs to adapt for use with providers.

Further information

Securing equity and excellence in commissioning specialised services, NHS Commissioning Board, November 2012.

Securing excellence in commissioning primary care, NHS Commissioning Board, June 2012.

Clinical commissioning groups' role

Through CCGs, GPs and other healthcare professionals – including nurses, allied health professionals and pharmacists – are responsible for commissioning most services to meet their patients' needs. CCGs commission:

- community health services
- maternity services
- elective hospital care
- urgent and emergency care, including ambulance and out-of-hours services
- older people's healthcare
- children's healthcare
- rehabilitation
- mental healthcare
- healthcare services for people with learning disabilities
- continuing healthcare
- infertility services.

A CCG may work in partnership with other CCGs or NHS England to commission certain services across a wider area or take part in major service reconfiguration. CCGs may also agree to commission some health improvement services jointly with local authorities. This could include, for example, obesity, smoking cessation and drug and alcohol services. They will have a duty to promote integrated health and social care. CCGs cannot delegate commissioning decisions to private companies or contractors. This does not prevent them from using external agencies for commissioning support (see page 32) such as data analysis.

The NHS Outcomes Framework (see page 80) specifies the outcomes for which CCGs are accountable. In planning services, CCGs will be involved in:

- identifying inequalities in access, quality and outcomes
- identifying indicators in the outcomes indicator set (see page 33) with scope for local improvement
- redesigning services or pathways to improve outcomes and better meet patients' needs
- identifying the most effective and cost-effective services, and planning new investments and disinvestments.

Every CCG must publish a commissioning plan before the start of each financial year, explaining how it intends to improve quality and outcomes, as well as fulfil its financial duties. In compiling this, the CCG must gather views from patients, carers, local communities, interest groups, health and wellbeing boards and local authorities. CCGs need to be able to translate individual patients' views into commissioning decisions, as well as act on the voice of each practice population. Their constituent practices should be significantly engaged, and they must also involve all other clinical colleagues – clinicians in secondary care, community and mental health, and learning disabilities, as well as public health experts and social care colleagues.

Once the plan is agreed, CCGs place contracts with providers for the services they wish to commission. They must monitor providers' performance against these contracts, particularly in relation to quality and outcomes, patient experience, clinical standards, activity levels and spending.

Although health professionals have overall responsibility for commissioning through their CCG, they are not expected to be involved in every commissioning function. Each CCG has a management allowance to enable it to buy in – or share with other organisations – specialist expertise to support the non-clinical aspects of commissioning. Commercial, local authority, third sector and other organisations offer commissioning support skills such as analysing population health needs, managing contracts with providers and monitoring expenditure and outcomes.

Further information
Everyone counts: planning for patients 2013/14, NHS Commissioning Board, December 2012.
The functions of clinical commissioning groups, DH, June 2012.

Commissioning support services (CSSs)
NHS England is temporarily hosting 19 commissioning support services from April 2013. Their role is to help CCGs by carrying out functions such as service redesign, market management, healthcare procurement, contract negotiation and monitoring, information analysis, and risk stratification. NHS England intends that CSSs become standalone enterprises by 2016. CCGs can choose where to secure the clinical support service they require. This may involve using its own staff, or purchasing the service from expert external organisations – which could be commercial, third sector or NHS.

Further information
Developing commissioning support: towards service excellence, NHS Commissioning Board, February 2012.

Contracting for services

The 2013/14 NHS standard contract, prepared by NHS England, covers all agreements between commissioners and providers of NHS-funded acute hospital, ambulance, community, mental health and learning disability services. Separate NHS standard contracts are available for care homes and high-security services.

The contract creates legally binding agreements between commissioners, local authorities, foundation trusts, social enterprises, independent and voluntary sector providers. Agreements between commissioners and NHS trusts are not legally binding, but use the same documents and are treated as if they were.

The contract provides a framework for holding providers to account for delivering NHS-funded services. It reflects the policy requirements such as patient choice (see page 45) and payment by results (see page 114).

Further information
The NHS standard contract: a guide for clinical commissioners, NHS Commissioning Board, February 2013.

Outcomes indicator set

The outcomes indicator set (formerly known as the Commissioning Outcomes Framework) measures the health outcomes and quality of care – including patient experience – achieved by CCGs. It has been developed by NHS England supported by NICE (see page 101), in consultation with professional and patient groups.

The indicators enable NHS England to identify CCGs' contribution to achieving the priorities for health improvement in the NHS Outcomes Framework (see page 80), while being accountable to patients and local communities. CCGs can also use it to benchmark their performance and identify priorities for improvement.

It comprises indicators in eight categories:
- cardiovascular
- gastrointestinal
- respiratory
- mental health
- endocrine, nutritional and metabolic
- maternity and reproductive
- cancer and tumours
- others/cross-cutting.

Further information
The CCG outcomes indicator set 2013/14: fact sheet, NHS Commissioning Board,
December 2012.

Health and wellbeing boards' role

Health and wellbeing boards (see page 19) assess local needs through joint
strategic needs assessments, and make collaborative decisions on how
best to meet those needs through a joint health and wellbeing strategy.
They also have a crucial role in promoting joint commissioning and
integrated provision of health, public health and social care services.

The aim is to ensure coherent and coordinated local commissioning plans
across the NHS, public health and social care – for example, in relation to
mental health, older people's or children's care, with intelligence about
needs systematically shaping commissioning decisions. Through the HWB,
councillors, public health directors and clinicians have critical roles to
play in the process.

HWBs should also be involved throughout development of CCGs'
commissioning plans, which are expected to align with the health and
wellbeing strategy. Though HWBs do not have a veto, they have a right
to refer plans back to the CCG or to NHS England if they think plans do
not take proper account of the strategy.

Joint strategic needs assessment

Joint strategic needs assessments (JSNAs) analyse populations' health
needs to inform and guide commissioning of health, wellbeing and social
care services within local authority areas. The NHS and upper-tier local
authorities have had a statutory duty to produce an annual JSNA since
2007. The JSNA now has a central role in bringing together organisations
from across the NHS, local government and the voluntary sector to

analyse health needs. It is an essential part of the commissioning cycle, guiding decisions made at every stage from strategic planning and service provision through to monitoring and evaluation. The Government believes HWBs will be able to take JSNAs further through collaborative leadership and development of joint health and wellbeing strategies.

Conducting a needs assessment involves a wide range of quantitative and qualitative data, including patient, user and community views, to produce a comprehensive picture of current and future health needs for adults and children. Specialist skills and resources are needed to capture, collate, analyse and interpret population-level data.

The product is intended to improve health and wellbeing outcomes, and help address persistent health inequalities. The JSNA should guide CCGs, the local authority and NHS England in deciding where to invest or reduce spending. Challenges may include integrating complex organisations with different agendas to agree on shared priorities, and organising CCGs that span several local authority areas to engage with the process.

Joint health and wellbeing strategy
To meet the needs outlined in its JSNA, each HWB must develop a joint health and wellbeing strategy, setting local priorities for joint action. This should enable the HWB to plan integrated local services, and can be used to influence wider determinants of health. It is also an opportunity for HWBs' constituent organisations to explore together local issues they have not managed to tackle on their own.

Joint health and wellbeing strategies provide the framework within which more detailed and specific commissioning plans for the NHS, social care, public health and other services are developed. Strategies should be 'concise and high-level', setting out how they will address a community's needs, rather than large, technical documents duplicating other plans.

Joint commissioning
The NHS and local government – in effect, CCGs and HWBs – will commission some services jointly. This should help integrate provision for patients, social care users and carers by connecting social care, public health and NHS services with aspects of the wider local authority agenda that affect health and wellbeing, such as housing and education.

HWBs can be the vehicle for 'lead commissioning' for particular services – for example, social care for people with long-term conditions – with pooled budgets and joint commissioning arrangements where the relevant functions are delegated to them. Tackling health inequalities is a major priority for HWBs.

Further information

Statutory guidance on joint strategic needs assessment and joint health and wellbeing strategies, DH, March 2013.

Operating principles for joint strategic needs assessments and joint health and wellbeing strategies: enabling joint decision-making for improved health and wellbeing, NHS Confederation and partners, November 2012.

Commissioning and competition

The Government says the NHS should use competition where it is in patients' interests, but it must also ensure integration and safeguard choice, quality and patient safety. Commissioners must uphold patients' rights to choice, but beyond that it is for them to decide if, when and how to use competition. However, they must act transparently and be able to demonstrate the rationale for their decisions.

The Health and Social Care Act 2012 sets the parameters on choice and competition within which Monitor and NHS England will work:
- Monitor must prevent anti-competitive behaviour that is against service users' interests
- NHS England must enable patients to make choices about services provided for them.

Fears that local services might be forced to use competition against patients' best interests led the Government to amend the NHS procurement, patient choice and competition regulations so that:
- there is no requirement to put all contracts out to competitive tender: commissioners are able to offer contracts to a single provider where only that provider is capable of providing the service
- Monitor has no power to force competitive tendering of services: decisions about how and when to introduce competition to improve services are solely up to CCGs
- competition should not trump integration: commissioners are free to commission an integrated service where it is in patients' interest.

Previously the regulations implied that commissioners could only award a contract without competition in very narrow circumstances. However, some commissioners remain concerned that this is still the case.

The regulations prohibit anti-competitive behaviour unless it is in patients' interests. 'Behaviour in the interests of patients' may include integrating services, or providers cooperating to improve service quality.

Monitor hosts the Cooperation and Competition Panel, which investigates potentially anti-competitive behaviour. Its approach is 'grounded in the established principles of economic and competition analysis', and its members have backgrounds in law, economics, business and healthcare.

Any proposed merger involving NHS foundation trusts will be reviewed by the Office of Fair Trading (OFT) to assess the impact on competition and whether or not the merger will operate in the interests of patients. Monitor will advise the OFT about the patient benefits of the proposed transaction. If the OFT decides that the merger might lead to a lessening of competition, and this outweighs any patient benefits of the transaction, it will refer the issue to the Competition Commission.

NHS England and Monitor are developing a 'choice and competition framework' to help commissioners decide how and when to use choice and competition to best effect.

Further information
Securing the best value for patients – consultation response document, DH, February 2013.
Choice and competition: delivering real choice, NHS Future Forum, June 2011.

Public health
Public health is concerned with improving the population's health, rather than treating the diseases of individual patients. Safeguarding and enhancing public health is therefore an important objective of commissioning. The official definition of public health, devised by former Chief Medical Officer Sir Donald Acheson, is: 'the science and art of preventing disease, prolonging life, and promoting health through the organised efforts of society'.

Public health comprises three 'domains':
• health improvement – including lifestyles, health inequalities and wider social influences on health
• health protection – including infectious diseases, environmental hazards and emergency preparedness
• health services – including service planning, efficiency, audit and evaluation.

Many of the aims of public health can only be achieved through partnerships across government departments and between the Government, NHS, local authorities, the private and voluntary sectors. This is especially true for tackling inequalities in health. Other major challenges include obesity, smoking, sexually transmitted diseases, alcohol and drug misuse and improving mental health.

Since 2013 local government rather than the NHS has had lead responsibility for public health. Its public health responsibilities already included environmental health, air quality, planning, transport and housing. Now upper-tier and unitary local authorities also have a legal duty to improve their population's health, with new powers and ringfenced budgets to help them do so.

Further information
Healthy lives, healthy people: update and way forward, HM Government, July 2011.

Public Health England

Public Health England (PHE) provides a national voice for public health, integrating health improvement, health protection and population health services into a single organisation.

An executive agency of the DH, PHE provides impartial advice to the Government, public and others, as well as providing advice, support, evidence and intelligence to local authorities and CCGs. It also provides microbiology and health protection services, and leads the public health response in emergencies. It works with the devolved administrations on UK-wide issues – for example, on chemical hazards and radiological protection.

Locally, PHE generates information on the state of public health in England to support development of JSNAs and joint health and wellbeing strategies (see page 34). It is also working with academic researchers and public health practitioners to build an evidence base of effective interventions, ensuring they share best practice and achieve value for money. It monitors local authorities' contributions to achieving the Public Health Outcomes Framework (see page 41).

PHE plays a key role in protecting people from hazards, including infectious diseases, radiation, chemicals and poisons, and any emergencies they cause.

PHE has a national office and operates through four regions and 15 centres.

Further information
Structure of Public Health England – factsheet, DH, July 2012.

Local authorities and public health

The Government says local authorities are best placed to tackle the wider determinants of health such as employment, education, environment, housing and transport, and so are a natural home for a public health function. Their new responsibilities include:

- tobacco control
- alcohol and drug misuse services
- obesity and community nutrition initiatives
- increasing physical activity
- public mental health services
- dental public health services
- accidental injury prevention
- population-level interventions to reduce and prevent birth defects
- campaigns to prevent cancer and long-term conditions
- local initiatives on workplace health
- supporting, reviewing and challenging NHS services such as immunisation programmes
- comprehensive sexual health services
- promoting community safety, violence prevention and response
- local initiatives to tackle social exclusion.

In addition, they are responsible for the National Child Measurement Programme, NHS Health Check assessment and elements of the Healthy Child Programme. Local authorities are funded to carry out their public health responsibilities through a ringfenced grant – just under £2.7 billion in 2013/14 and just under £2.8 billion in 2014/15. Within local authorities, HWBs are envisaged as the focus of the public health system, promoting joint commissioning and driving improvements in the local population's health and wellbeing (see page 34).

Further information
Local public health intelligence – factsheets, DH, September 2012.

NHS and public health

The NHS's role in securing population health outcomes includes:
- providing healthcare to meet the local population's needs
- providing population health interventions such as childhood immunisations and national screening programmes
- contributing to health protection and emergency response.

If the NHS uses its millions of contacts with patients every year to provide advice, brief interventions and referrals, it can make an impact on public health by supporting people to live healthier lives. The NHS will also continue to play an important role in commissioning and providing public health services.

Further information
The NHS's role in the public's health: a report from the NHS Future Forum, DH, January 2012.

Secretary of State's role

The Secretary of State's responsibilities for public health include:
- setting a ringfenced budget for public health from within the overall health budget
- setting the direction for PHE and the context for local public health efforts
- leading public health across central government, through the cabinet subcommittee on public health
- setting the national Public Health Outcomes Framework (see opposite)
- holding PHE to account
- leading public health work across civil society and business, and brokering national partnerships
- participating in public health work across the UK with the devolved administrations and at European and international levels
- proposing legislation where necessary
- commissioning research for public health.

Further information
The new public health system: summary, DH, December 2011.

Key text: Public Health Outcomes Framework

The Public Health Outcomes Framework concentrates on two goals to be achieved across the public health system:
• increased healthy life expectancy
• reduced differences in life expectancy and healthy life expectancy between communities.

As improvements will take years or decades before marked change is evident, 66 supporting indicators will measure national and local progress annually across four domains:
• improving the wider determinants of health
• health improvement
• health protection
• healthcare public health and preventing premature mortality.

Progress will be judged against results such as:
• fewer children under five with tooth decay
• people weighing less
• more women breastfeeding their babies
• fewer people over 65 suffering falls
• fewer people smoking
• fewer people dying from heart disease and stroke.

Further information
Improving outcomes and supporting transparency – part 1A: a public health outcomes framework for England 2013–2016, DH, November 2012.
Improving outcomes and supporting transparency – public health outcomes framework factsheet, DH, November 2012.

03 Providing services

NHS organisations provide a wide range of services, outside hospitals and within them. Historically, hospitals have dominated the NHS's resources, but today much more care can be provided in GP surgeries and health centres closer to people's homes – and it is government policy that it should be. It wants patients to have much more choice than hitherto over where they are treated, and it wants the services provided to feel more personal, taking greater account of people's preferences than was customary in the past.

Primary care

Primary care is normally the patient's first point of consultation with the health service. It is concerned with promoting health as well as treating and managing conditions that do not require specialist care in hospital. For NHS patients, primary care provides the key to navigating the rest of the healthcare system. GPs, community nurses, health visitors, allied health professionals, pharmacists, dentists and opticians have a role as advocates for patients needing services from other parts of the NHS. Providing continuity of care is another important aspect.

About 90 per cent of NHS patients receive their treatment in primary care, and over 300 million consultations take place every year in England alone. Advances, especially in diagnostics and minor surgery, mean many more treatments once carried out in hospital can be performed in primary care – a rapidly growing trend convenient for patients and of benefit to the system as a whole. Over 5 million people in England live more than ten miles from their nearest hospital.

A wide range of staff work in primary care in England. In 2012 there were:
• 40,265 GPs
• 23,458 practice nurses
• 113,832 practice staff, including practice managers, receptionists, IT support and notes summarisers, physiotherapists, podiatrists, counsellors, phlebotomists and healthcare assistants.

General practitioners

Most GP practices are independent contractors (see page 26) and are run as partnerships, while specialist companies run some practices. The number of practices has fallen in recent years although the number of GPs has increased, suggesting practices have become bigger.

Under the general medical services contract, all GP practices are required to provide 'essential services': they must manage patients who are ill or

patient choice

Since 2009 patients referred for an elective procedure have had a legal right under the NHS Constitution to choose any hospital, clinic or treatment centre in England which meets NHS standards and price, including those in the independent sector. Since 2012, patients have had the right to choose a hospital consultant-led team for a first outpatient appointment for elective care. No geographical boundaries are imposed on referrals, and NHS providers must publish relevant information about their consultants and the services they provide. Patients can also choose where to undergo a medical test if referred for one by their GP.

To help choose a provider, patients can use a national directory of services that is part of the Choose and Book facility on the NHS Choices website (see page 48), which also lets them choose a time and date for their appointment. Information includes location, waiting times, reputation, clinical performance, visiting policies, parking facilities and other patients' comments.

Choose and Book is currently used for more than 50 per cent of NHS referral activity from GP surgery to first outpatient appointment – more than 500,000 appointments a month plus another 150,000 a month for services offered by allied health professionals (see page 49). More than 30 million appointments have been booked using Choose and Book and more than 95 per cent of all GP practices have used it to refer patients.

Further information
2013/14 choice framework, DH, December 2012.
NHS Choices **www.nhs.uk**
Choose and Book **www.chooseandbook.nhs.uk**

believe themselves to be ill, giving health promotion advice and making referrals as necessary. They must also manage patients who are terminally ill and those with chronic diseases. All practices may provide 'additional services' such as contraception or childhood immunisations, but they can opt out of them. They may also choose to provide 'enhanced services' in response to need, such as identifying and managing seriously ill patients or those at risk of emergency hospital admission. The Quality and Outcomes Framework (see page 76) is designed to maintain high standards and broaden the range of services GPs offer.

The Government is keen for GPs to widen their role to include services traditionally found only in hospitals. It believes that those with accredited specialist skills could handle more minor operations, while specially trained GPs and senior consultants should routinely work together in community hospitals and health centres. Operations for conditions such as cataracts, hernia and varicose veins can be done on the same site, reducing waiting times and potentially saving money.

The 2012 GP patient survey found:
- 92.8 per cent of patients have confidence and trust in their doctor
- 87.6 per cent of patients rate their overall experience of their GP practice as good
- 80.5 per cent of patients are satisfied with their surgery opening hours.

Further information
GP patient survey results **www.gp-patient.co.uk**

Dental services
Most dentists in primary care are self-employed and contract their services to the NHS, like most GPs. They numbered 22,920 in 2011/12.

Access to dentistry has been a high-profile issue for 20 years, with concerns about gaps in access to NHS-funded services and practices opting out or closing to new NHS patients. Policy on dental services lagged behind other health sectors until 2006, when over 400 charges for treatment were replaced by three standard charges for all treatments under a revised dental contract. The budget for primary care dental services was devolved to commissioners, and covered surgery salaries and expenses instead of the piecework pay system set up when the NHS was founded. However, the 2006 contract did not succeed in incentivising preventive care rather than focusing on a fee-per-item approach, and dentists widely perceived it as unfair.

A new dental contract is now being piloted in 98 practices, structured to reward dentists for continuity and quality of care rather than the number of treatments undertaken. It is based on registration, capitation and quality. Its aim is to improve care quality, increase access to dental services and improve oral health, especially children's.

The Office of Fair Trading called for patients to be given better information about their choice of dentist and treatment: it found about 500,000 patients a year were given inaccurate information by their dentist about treatments they are entitled to on the NHS and as a result paid to receive private treatment.

Further information
Government response to the Office of Fair Trading market study into dentistry, HM Government, August 2012.

Community pharmacies
England's 11,236 high street pharmacies dispensed 885 million prescription items in 2011/12. They increasingly offer services traditionally available only at GPs' surgeries. The pharmacy contract introduced in 2005 aims to improve the range and quality of services of the community pharmacy and integrate it more into the NHS. It defines three tiers of service:
- Essential services must be provided by all community pharmacists. They include dispensing, disposal of medication and support for self-care.
- Advanced services require the pharmacist to have accreditation and/or their premises to meet certain standards. So far, medicines use review and prescription intervention fall into this category.
- Enhanced services are commissioned locally. Examples include minor ailment schemes and smoking-cessation services.

Many pharmacies now offer new services such as:
- repeat prescribing, so that patients can get up to a year's supply of medicines without having to revisit their GP
- clinics for people with conditions such as diabetes, high blood pressure or high cholesterol
- signposting other health and social care services and supporting self-care
- consultation areas.

Opticians
There were 11,133 ophthalmic practitioners in England in 2012, and 12.3 million NHS eye tests were carried out. There are three kinds of registered optician:

Optometrists – or ophthalmic opticians – carry out eye tests, look for signs of eye disease and prescribe and fit glasses and contact lenses. They are graduates who have undertaken a three- or four-year degree in optometry, then spent at least a year in supervised practice before taking professional exams leading to registration with the General Optical Council. There were 10,829 registered optometrists in England in 2012.

Dispensing opticians fit and sell glasses, and interpret prescriptions but do not test eyes. Some dispense low-vision aids, and some are qualified to fit contact lenses under instruction from an optometrist.

Ophthalmic medical practitioners practitioners are doctors specialising in eyes and eye care. There were 304 in England in 2012. They work to the same terms of service as optometrists.

In addition, ophthalmologists are doctors specialising in eye diseases and most perform eye surgery. They usually work in hospital eye departments. Orthoptists treat disorders of binocular vision, and work in eye departments under the supervision of ophthalmologists. They may also undertake visual screening of children in the community. Some GPs have a special interest in ophthalmology, while ophthalmic nurses and ophthalmic technicians – or ophthalmic science practitioners – also provide services.

Optometrists are independent contractors. Some have specialist skills – for example, in contact lenses, low vision or paediatrics – and can treat patients who would otherwise have to be seen in hospital. Most practices have much of the equipment found in ophthalmology clinics.

Under co-management, or shared care, optometrists working to an agreed protocol undertake specified clinical procedures designed to relieve GPs and the hospital eye service, as well as move patient care into the community. This may cover conditions such as glaucoma, diabetes, cataracts and minor acute eye problems. Throughout the UK, optometrists can now prescribe medicines for conditions of the eye and surrounding tissue if they are registered to do so with the General Optical Council and have undertaken special training.

Community health services

Community health services are a major part of the NHS, employing 250,000 people and costing over £11 billion a year. They provide a wide range of care, from supporting people with long-term conditions to treating patients with complex illnesses. Historically they have often been overlooked by policymakers, but they are well placed to play a central role in achieving many of the aims of NHS reform, such as providing more personalised care closer to patients' homes, helping avoid unnecessary hospital admissions or shortening hospital stays, as well as leading efforts on preventive and wellness services. They also offer preventive and health improvement services, often in partnership with local government and the third sector.

A variety of staff and organisations provide a range of health services in the community.

Allied health professionals – Qualified AHPs number about 75,000 and form a diverse group of statutory-registered practitioners who include art therapists, drama therapists, music therapists, chiropodists/podiatrists, dietitians, occupational therapists, orthoptists, orthotists and prosthetists, paramedics, physiotherapists, diagnostic radiographers, therapeutic radiographers and speech and language therapists. In recent years the DH has encouraged AHPs to accept patients who refer themselves to AHP services.

Community nurses – who include district nurses with a post-registration qualification, registered nurses and healthcare assistants. More than half the patients they see will be aged over 75. About half their work comes from GP referrals and a quarter from hospital staff; patients and carers can also refer themselves.

Community matrons – as experienced nurses, community matrons use case management techniques with patients who make intensive use of healthcare to help them remain at home longer. They numbered 1,469 in 2012.

Health visitors – who are registered nurses or midwives with additional training and experience in child health, health promotion and education. Much of their work is with mothers and babies using a child-centred, family-focused approach, although they do provide more general health advice to people of all ages. Their support staff include nursery nurses and healthcare assistants, who focus on less complex family support and parenting skills. The Government plans to recruit an extra 4,200 health visitors by 2015. They numbered 10,227 in 2012.

Midwives – generally attached to hospitals, but working in both hospital and community settings. They numbered 25,654 in 2012.

Specialist nurses – with expertise in a variety of specialisms including stoma care, continence services, palliative care and support for people with long-term conditions.

A wide range of other health-related services come under the umbrella of community health:

School nursing – providing support and advice to school-age children, their parents and schools on health issues, a role which has evolved considerably in recent years. School nurses numbered 1,498 in 2012.

Community dentistry and dental public health – providing services to schools and people with a variety of special needs.

Podiatry – foot care for elderly people or those with diabetes, gait or lower limb problems. Independent contractors provide much of this care. More than half the service is for people aged over 65.

Physiotherapy – sometimes provided by GP practices or hospitals in a community setting, with emphasis on rehabilitation.

Occupational therapy – providing advice, aids and adaptations. Some staff specialise in adults, some in children. The service is often provided by other agencies, such as local government, although in some cases the NHS provides local authority OT services.

Speech and language therapy – services for children and adults who have difficulty with communicating, eating, drinking or swallowing.

Clinical psychology – often provided by specialist mental health trusts, although more than 40 per cent of referrals come from general practice.

Family planning services – may cover sexual health problems as well as contraception, vasectomy and termination clinics and specialist clinics for young people.

Community rehabilitation – often for stroke or cardiac conditions. Services may be delivered by specialist teams in the patient's home or by combining intermediate care or community hospital care with home care.

Further information
Briefing 258: Transforming local care: community healthcare rises to the challenge, NHS
Confederation, March 2013.

Integrated care

Integrated care involves health and social care services working together.
Demographic change means more people are living with long-term or
multiple health problems: those with physical and learning disabilities,
carers and multi-agency support for children all demand more integrated
care, and there is an expectation that once-fragmented services can be
coordinated to provide person-centred care that facilitates earlier and
more cost-effective interventions.

On the front line, integrated care means GPs, community nurses,
pharmacists, social care teams, ambulance services, schools, patient
groups and others working collaboratively with clear leadership, shared
goals and shared information, and designing services around the needs
of individuals and local communities.

Integration is especially important for continuing care, long-term care,
intermediate care and end-of-life care, which – to be effective – all
depend on a high degree of coordination between different organisations.
Integration might involve bringing together different kinds of expertise
and interventions – for example, by creating teams of primary and
secondary care clinicians, or health and social care professionals.

Some policy analysts have questioned whether integrating services is
compatible with increasing competition in the NHS. Others argue that
examples from western Europe suggest it is possible with sound
commissioning arrangements in place. Among the principles that some
argue must be observed to make integrated care a reality are: giving
patients more control over their care packages; focusing integrated
services on patient groups most in need; ensuring health and social care
leaders jointly deliver locally appropriate solutions; and developing
incentives to reward organisations that achieve integrated care.

NHS England and the Local Government Association (LGA) have signed
a concordat to work together to better integrate health and social care.
They will produce joint annual plans setting out how they intend to do
this, assess progress and set future priorities.

Further information
Making integrated out-of-hospital care a reality, NHS Confederation/Royal College of GPs, December 2012.
Concordat between: Local Government Association and NHS Commissioning Board, LGA/NHSCB, October 2012.
Briefing 240: A stitch in time – the future is integration, NHS Confederation, June 2012.

Integrated care pilot programme
The DH launched a £4 million programme involving 16 pilots in 2009 to test different models of integrated care. The sites involved partnerships of primary care with social care, secondary care, and the voluntary and private sectors. Issues examined included dementia, care for the elderly, substance misuse, chronic obstructive pulmonary disease and end-of-life care. The methods involved included partnerships, new systems and care pathways that span primary, community, secondary and social care. Independent evaluation found that integration was most likely to improve healthcare processes but less likely to improve patient experience or to reduce costs, at least in the short term. Its impact on reducing demand for emergency hospital care varies according to local factors.

Further information
National evaluation of the Department of Health's integrated care pilots: final report, RAND Europe and Ernst & Young, March 2012.

Continuing healthcare
Continuing healthcare is care provided over an extended period to someone aged 18 or over to meet physical and mental health needs that have arisen as a result of disability, accident or illness. The person may require services from the NHS and/or local authorities. Where they are assessed as having mainly health needs, the NHS will arrange and fund the complete package, which may be provided in any setting – hospital, hospice, home or care home. If they live in a care home, the NHS will contribute to their nursing care. Eligibility for NHS continuing healthcare is based on needs, not ability to pay. If a person does not qualify, the NHS may still have responsibility for contributing to a 'joint package' to meet their health needs.

About 56,000 people received NHS continuing healthcare in 2012/13, costing £2.5 billion a year.

Further information
Briefing 256: NHS continuing healthcare: detailing what NHS organisations need to know and do, NHS Confederation, November 2012.
National framework for NHS continuing healthcare and NHS-funded nursing care (revised), DH, November 2012.

Care for long-term conditions
More than 17.5 million people in the UK (15.4 million in England) suffer a long-term or chronic condition such as diabetes, asthma or arthritis. They represent more than 50 per cent of GP appointments, 65 per cent of outpatient appointments and accident and emergency attendances, and more than 70 per cent of inpatient admissions. In total, they account for around 70 per cent of total health and social care spend, according to the DH. Their numbers are forecast to increase by 252 per cent by 2050.

Best practice requires early recognition, prompt diagnosis and treatment, early and specialist rehabilitation, equipment and accommodation and support for family and carers. For best quality care – and to maximise service efficiency – it is important that long-term conditions are effectively managed outside hospital wherever possible.

Health and social care organisations should assign 'community matrons' (see page 49) to the most vulnerable patients with complex multiple long-term conditions to monitor them, anticipate any problems and coordinate their care. Multi-professional teams should identify all people with a single serious long-term illness, assess their needs as early as possible and provide proactive care before their condition deteriorates. Everyone with a long-term condition should be educated about their health and encouraged to manage their own care more effectively.

Everyone with a long-term condition should be offered a personalised care plan. These address an individual's full range of needs, taking into account their health, personal, family, social, economic, educational, mental health, ethnic and cultural background and circumstances. The plan can be a written document or electronically recorded or recorded in the person's notes and accessible to them.

older people's health

Older people are the main users of the NHS: although they make up about a fifth of the population, they occupy two-thirds of hospital beds, and are three times more likely to be admitted to hospital.

Reports suggest older people do not always receive the same standard of care from the NHS as younger patients. But since the Equality Act 2010 came into force in 2012, arbitrary and harmful age discrimination in the NHS has been banned, including:

- making assumptions about whether an older patient should be referred for treatment based solely on their age, rather than on need
- not referring certain age groups for a particular treatment that is considered mainly – but not exclusively – for working-age adults
- not considering the wellbeing or dignity of older people.

Commissioners and providers of NHS and social care services may continue to make clinically justifiable decisions based on age for relevant services such as eligibility for screening and vaccination programmes. The Act aims to prevent only harmful discrimination, not discrimination for which there are beneficial or justifiable reasons.

There are currently 650,000 people with dementia in England, and by 2025 it is expected that over 1 million people in the UK will be living with dementia. The National Audit Office estimates that dementia costs health and social care services £8.2 billion a year. Every general hospital has excess costs of £6 million because of the condition, due to worse outcomes for length of stay, mortality and institutionalisation.

In 2012 the Prime Minister launched the 'dementia challenge' with the aim of: creating dementia-friendly communities that understand how to help; driving improvements in health and care; and improving research. A range of related initiatives have followed, including a £50 million fund to create areas in care homes and hospitals that help to reduce anxiety and distress in people with dementia, and £9.6 million for dementia research.

Further information

The Prime Minister's challenge on dementia – delivering major improvements in dementia care and research by 2015: a report on progress, DH, November 2012.

Delivering dignity: securing dignity in care for older people in hospitals and care homes, NHS Confederation/LGA/Age UK, June 2012.

Dementia Challenge http://dementiachallenge.dh.gov.uk

The 2012 NHS Mandate (see page 18) instructs NHS England to devise plans to improve life for people with long-term conditions by:
- helping them acquire skills to manage their own health
- agreeing with them a care plan based on their personal needs
- ensuring their care is better coordinated.

Further information
Long term conditions compendium of information: third edition, DH, May 2012.
Investing in emotional and psychological wellbeing for patients with long-term conditions, NHS Confederation, April 2012.
Improving care for people with long term conditions: information sheet 1 – personalised care planning, an 'at a glance' guide for healthcare professionals, DH, February 2011.

Self-care
The DH devised seven core principles of self-care to help health and social care staff support people with long-term conditions or complex needs to live independently and stay healthy. They are:
- ensure people can make informed choices to manage their self-care needs
- communicate effectively to enable people to assess their needs and gain confidence to care for themselves
- support and enable people to access appropriate information to manage their self-care
- support and enable individuals to develop skills in self-care
- support and enable individuals to use technology for self-care
- advise individuals how to access support networks and participate in planning, developing and evaluating services
- support and enable risk management and risk-taking to maximise independence and choice.

A networking and resource website, Self Care Connect, is run by the Expert Patients Programme for those with a professional interest in self-care.

The Self Care Forum was set up in 2011 with the aim of 'furthering the reach of self-care and embedding it into everyday life'. Members include patients, GPs, nurses, pharmacists, health service managers and the DH. The forum organises a national self-care week annually.

Further information
Improving care for people with long term conditions: information sheet 5 – what motivates people to self care, an 'at a glance' guide for healthcare professionals, DH, February 2011.
Self Care Connect www.selfcareconnect.co.uk
Self Care Forum www.selfcareforum.org

End-of-life care

Half a million people die in England each year, three-quarters after a chronic illness. Surveys show most people would prefer to die at home: in 2011 there were 21.8 per cent who did so; 51 per cent died in hospital, 19.4 per cent in care homes, about 4 per cent in a hospice and 3 per cent elsewhere. End-of-life care is becoming more complex, with people living longer and the incidence of frailty and multiple conditions in older people rising. The DH therefore launched a ten-year end-of-life care strategy in 2008 to help more people to die in the setting they choose, to promote dignity and respect, and to properly coordinate services and support carers.

It focuses on:
- improved community services, ensuring rapid-response community nursing services are available everywhere around the clock
- workforce training and development in assessing patients' and carers' needs and providing best-quality care
- developing specialist palliative care outreach services in the community, to support all adults regardless of their condition
- setting up a national end-of-life research initiative on how best to care for those at the end of their lives
- quality standards against which commissioners and providers can assess themselves and be assessed by regulators.

The National End-of-Life Care Programme aims to support implementation of the strategy by sharing good practice, and is backed with £286 million of government money. The first National Bereavement Survey in 2011 found 75 per cent rated end-of-life care positively, while 92 per cent rated hospice care as excellent or good.

Further information

End of life care strategy – fourth annual report, DH, October 2012.
Funding the right care and support for everyone: creating a fair and transparent funding system; the final report of the palliative care funding review, Palliative Care Funding Review, July 2011.
Improving care for people with long term conditions: information sheet 8 – end of life care and personalised care planning, an 'at a glance' guide for healthcare professionals, DH, February 2011.

personal health budgets

Personal health budgets are designed to enhance independence and choice for people receiving care or support. A personal budget combines resources from different funding streams into a single sum. The purpose is to give people a clear idea of the finance available and enable them to make their own decisions about their care – for example, by having someone support them at home rather than going into residential care.

The care plan – setting out the individual's health and social care needs, desired outcomes, money available and how it will be spent – is at the heart of the personal health budget. It is developed by the patient and/or their carer in partnership with their healthcare professionals and others, then agreed with the clinical commissioning group. The amount of money in the budget and what it can be spent on is decided according to the individual's needs.

After pilot schemes that ran from 2009, personal health budgets are now being implemented nationally for the 56,000 people receiving NHS continuing healthcare (see page 52). People with a range of long-term conditions such as stroke, diabetes, neurological conditions, mental health needs and respiratory problems were involved in the pilots.

Evaluation of the pilots found that personal health budgets improved people's quality of life, though their health status stayed the same. Benefits were more marked where people had higher levels of need. Budgets also worked better where people were given more choice and control, both over what they bought and how they received the budget; where the pilot site imposed restrictions, personal health budgets tended to worsen people's outcomes.

Social care users have had personal budgets for many years, and a joint system between local authorities and the NHS could offer a new model for integrating care.

Further information

Evaluation of the personal health budget pilot programme, DH, November 2012.
Briefing 251: Joint personal budgets: a new solution to the problems of integrated care?
NHS Confederation, October 2012.
www.personalhealthbudgets.england.nhs.uk

Secondary care

The changing role of hospitals

Acute hospitals have always dominated healthcare spending and provision, but their role has begun to change fundamentally. Demographic, economic and technological changes are fuelling a drive to use community settings for some services traditionally provided in hospitals, in a way that emphasises support for health and wellbeing rather than simply curing disease.

Changes in the last two decades have revolutionised surgery: lasers and 'keyhole' techniques have led to quicker recovery and less risk of infection. Procedures that previously required long stays in hospital, such as hernia operations, can now be done as day cases more locally. Between 2000 and 2010 average lengths of stay in UK hospitals dropped by 27 per cent from 10.5 to 7.7 days. New drugs have made some surgery, such as treatment for stomach ulcers, completely unnecessary. Eighty per cent of all surgery could be done locally, leaving the most complex 20 per cent for specialist centres with the most highly skilled surgeons using the latest technology.

Meanwhile, patient choice, payment by results and the reorganisation of commissioning are affecting the balance of power between organisations, stimulating further change – especially as value for money has become even more important with the slowdown in spending (see page 118).

The result of these developments is that the traditional model of the district general hospital is changing. Local hospitals are likely to remain important, but rather than working in isolation will have to collaborate with other providers and each other as part of healthcare groups or networks. Rather than exercising local monopolies, hospitals will need to promote competition and choice.

Change to local health services is often controversial for staff and the public, who need to be involved in developing plans from early on. Proposals must demonstrate:
• support from clinical commissioners
• strengthened public and patient engagement
• clarity on the clinical evidence base
• consistency with current and prospective patient choice
• transparency and accountability in decision-making.

These tests are designed to ensure service changes are driven by local
clinicians, patients and their representatives.

Treatment centres

Treatment centres are units that carry out planned surgery and treatment
in areas that have traditionally had the longest waiting times, separating
them from unplanned care and so lessening the risk of cancelled
operations. They have developed new staff roles, including perioperative
specialist practitioners, advanced nurse practitioners/advisers and
healthcare assistant technicians in radiology, ophthalmology and surgery.

A treatment centre's essential features include:
• delivering a high volume of routine treatments and/or diagnostics
• streamlined services using defined pathways
• planned and booked services, with emphasis on patient choice
  and convenience.

Some are run by the NHS, others by the independent sector under contract
to the NHS. Centres may care for patients within a single specialty or a
range of specialties. The type of work they do falls into three categories:
• short-stay inpatient work, often in a single specialty such as
  orthopaedics or ophthalmology
• day-case or outpatient work
• community-based diagnostic work, such as endoscopy and ultrasound,
  and minor surgical procedures such as excision of cysts and lesions,
  and vasectomies.

Urgent and emergency care

The system for delivering urgent and emergency care includes:

- community pharmacy and self-care
- GP services, including out-of-hours services
- urgent care centres, including walk-in centres and minor injuries units
- ambulance services
- hospital accident and emergency departments
- critical care services.

Urgent care is for patients who have an injury or illness that requires immediate attention but is not usually serious enough to require a visit to an accident and emergency department.

NHS England is reviewing urgent and emergency care services after concerns that the system was becoming complex and fragmented amid rising demand. Although treatment for many common conditions such as heart attacks and strokes is best provided in specialist centres, the public want accident and emergency departments close by. The review will also examine proposals for more seven-day services.

111 – the national number for non-emergency care

A new, free telephone service, available by dialling 111, is providing access to urgent but non-emergency healthcare in the same way the existing 999 service enables instant access to emergency care.

Available 24 hours a day, the 111 service assesses callers' needs and provides clinical advice or information, or routes them to a local service such as a walk-in centre or minor injuries unit. If a caller needs to see a nurse or needs an urgent home visit in the middle of the night, NHS 111 will organise that. In the event of a caller needing emergency treatment, an ambulance is sent without the need for further assessment.

NHS 111 content is being made available online, including health information, checklists of symptoms and a directory of local services. A mobile phone app will offer the same services. GPs will be able to link their own booking systems to 111, allowing their patients to book an urgent appointment. The service is staffed by call advisers, supported by nurses.

The service is intended to be fully operational throughout England during 2013.

Ambulance services

Ambulance services have changed significantly in the past decade, with big improvements in response times for 999 calls, in training and quality of care, vehicle standards, equipment and technology. As demand for ambulances has risen steadily every year, ambulance services have developed to provide more diagnosis, treatment and care in people's homes, helping avoid unnecessary A&E admissions.

In addition to transporting patients, ambulance services now have a multiplicity of roles:

- helping patients access the most appropriate NHS services – call handlers must assess emergency calls and redirect callers to other services if necessary, as many people dial 999 unaware of how to access more appropriate non-emergency services
- taking care to the patient, not always taking the patient to hospital – only 70 per cent of patients treated by the ambulance service are taken to A&E, with the remainder often treated at home by paramedics
- promoting public health – including provision of first-aid training to local industry and campaigns raising awareness of the symptoms of serious illnesses
- preventing accidents – particularly reducing falls among older people by working with social care services
- safeguarding vulnerable children and adults – more than any other NHS service, ambulance crews operate in people's homes and have developed processes to ensure the right agencies receive the right referral, with all information treated confidentially and sensitively
- working with the local community – for example, by training local first responders to provide life-saving treatment like defibrillation while an ambulance is on its way, especially in rural areas.

Crews now use satellite navigation systems, and emergency ambulances are equipped with technology such as ECG machines and telemetry, which lets crews send information about a patient's condition directly to the receiving hospital. Services deploy solo responders, such as motorcycles and rapid-response vehicles, to travel through heavy traffic more easily.

Ambulance services are improving their ability to assess, diagnose and treat patients over the telephone and face to face. For example, new critical care paramedics – authorised to use pain-relief drugs and with enhanced resuscitation skills – are improving care for critically ill and injured patients.

Emergency care practitioners (ECPs) assess, diagnose and treat minor illnesses and injuries in the community or in people's homes, helping reduce unnecessary A&E admissions. ECPs also support GPs in and out of hours by making home visits. In parts of the country, ambulance services coordinate a single point of access to urgent care, ensuring patients get the most appropriate services for their clinical need.

Accident and emergency

About 20 million visits are made to A&E departments in England every year, and about one-fifth result in admissions to hospital as emergencies. Before a patient is admitted for further care, transferred or discharged, there can often be a lengthy chain of decisions, tests and treatment that can be subject to delay. From 2004 until 2011 A&E departments had a target of seeing, diagnosing and treating all patients within four hours of their arrival. This has now been replaced with a range of clinical quality standards to reflect timeliness and effectiveness of treatment – and overall patient experience – rather than focus solely on faster care. These include:

• unplanned re-attendance
• left without being seen
• total time spent in A&E
• time to initial assessment
• time to treatment.

Trauma services

Major trauma – severe injury including head injury – is the main cause of death in people under 40 and a cause of long-term disability. As it constitutes only a small proportion of acute activity – on average about two per hospital per week – it historically received relatively little management and planning attention. A series of critical reports from the Royal Colleges and others showed that services were inadequate. An estimated 450 to 600 lives could be saved in NHS hospitals every year if trauma services were better organised.

Therefore the NHS is establishing a network of 20 major trauma centres to ensure patients with serious and life-threatening injuries are treated quickly in a specialist hospital. They offer a full range of trauma specialists, including orthopaedics, neurosurgery and radiology teams. Care is led by a trauma consultant available 24 hours a day. Many patients need a personalised rehabilitation programme taking many months and involving physiotherapists, occupational and speech therapists, either at the major trauma centre or at other units in the area.

Critical care

Critical care comprises intensive and high-dependence care services and is provided to more than 300,000 patients annually in England. During the past decade a modernisation programme for critical care has integrated services for critically ill patients wherever they are in the health system. Key objectives were to:

- increase capacity
- develop services supporting critically ill patients throughout the hospital – not necessarily restricted to critical care 'units'
- provide an integrated critical care organisation within and between hospitals working in collaborative networks
- provide comprehensive information and data on critical care.

Maternity services

The NHS is striving to offer a wider choice of type and place of maternity care and birth. Services should be accessible to all women and be designed to take full account of their individual needs, including different language, cultural, religious and social needs or particular needs related to disability, including learning disability.

Four national 'choice guarantees' were introduced in 2009 so that all women can choose:

- how to access maternity care – by going straight to a midwife or a GP
- type of antenatal care – either midwifery or care provided by a team of maternity health professionals, including midwives and obstetricians
- place of birth – either at home, supported by a midwife; in a local midwifery unit or birth centre, which might be in the community or in a hospital, supported by a midwife; or in a hospital supported by a maternity team that may include midwives, obstetricians, paediatricians and anaesthetists
- postnatal care – either at home or in a community setting, such as a Sure Start children's centre.

The NHS Information Service for Parents is available to all new parents with a baby up to six months old. In 2012 the Government earmarked £25 million to improve maternity facilities.
www.nhs.uk/InformationServiceForParents

Mental health

At least one in four people will experience a mental health problem at some point in their life, and one in six adults has a mental health problem at any one time. Almost half of all adults will experience at least one episode of depression during their lifetime, while about one in 100 people has a severe mental illness. One in ten children aged between five and 16 years has a mental health problem. Mental health services absorb about 12 per cent of the NHS budget, while the number of consultant psychiatrists, clinical psychologists and mental health nurses has risen significantly in the last 15 years.

Today, the principles guiding mental healthcare are:
• care provided closer to home
• earlier intervention
• 24/7 home treatment
• care tailored to individuals' needs
• better access to modern drugs
• care provided by multi-disciplinary teams
• more use of talking therapies.

Further information
Factsheet: Key facts and trends in mental health – updated figures and statistics, Mental Health Network/NHS Confederation, September 2011.

Organising mental health services
Mental health services are provided as part of primary and secondary care by the NHS, social care and the independent and voluntary sectors. Provision comprises acute inpatient care, community and rehabilitation services, residential care centres, day hospitals and drop-in centres. About 80,000 staff work in statutory mental health services, and 1.2 million people are in contact with mental health services annually.

Further information
Briefing 253: Mental health and the market, NHS Confederation, October 2012.
Defining mental health services: promoting effective commissioning and supporting QIPP, NHS Confederation, January 2012.

A cross-government, all-age strategy for mental health in England was published in early 2011. *No health without mental health* stresses the Government's expectation that there be 'parity of esteem' between mental and physical health services. It has two underlying aims:
• to improve mental health and wellbeing and keep people well
• to improve outcomes through high-quality services equally accessible to all.

The strategy sets out six objectives:
• more people will have good mental health
• more people with mental health problems will recover
• more people with mental health problems will have good physical health
• more people will have a positive experience of care and support
• fewer people will suffer avoidable harm
• fewer people will experience stigma and discrimination.

It also includes commitments to:
• agree and use a new national measure of wellbeing
• challenge stigma
• ensure people in contact with the criminal justice system have improved access to mental health services
• launch a set of 'recovery' pilots to test the key features of organisational practice to support the recovery of those using mental health services.

A suicide-prevention strategy has also been published.

Further information
Preventing suicide in England: a cross-government outcomes strategy to save lives, HM Government, September 2012.
No health without mental health: implementation framework, DH and partners, July 2012.
No health without mental health: a cross-government mental health outcomes strategy for people of all ages, HM Government, February 2011.

Primary and community services

Of people who receive help for mental health problems – whether for depression, anxiety or other mental disorders, or for a psychotic illness such as schizophrenia – 90 per cent are dealt with in primary care: 30 per cent of GP consultations have a significant mental health component. GPs usually refer patients they cannot help directly to the local community mental health team (CMHT) or to a psychiatric outpatient clinic.

CMHTs provide community-based services for people with mental health problems. Everyone seen by specialist mental health services should have their need for treatment assessed, a care plan drawn up and a named mental health worker to coordinate their care, including a regular review of their needs. CMHTs aim to help provide continuity of care across different services, promote multi-professional and inter-agency working, and ensure appropriate care for people diagnosed with serious mental illness on discharge from hospital.

CMHT members include community psychiatric nurses, social workers, psychologists, occupational therapists, doctors and support workers.

Providing mental health services in the community has prompted new approaches to care to avoid hospital admission. For example:
• early intervention teams aim to treat psychotic illness as quickly and effectively as possible, especially during the critical period after its onset
• assertive outreach teams provide intensive support for severely mentally ill people who are difficult to engage in more traditional services
• home treatment and crisis resolution teams provide flexible acute care in patients' own homes with a 24-hour service to help with crises.

The availability of 'talking treatments' is being extended through the Improving Access to Psychological Therapies (IAPT) programme. This comprises:
• cognitive behavioural therapy (CBT)
• counselling for depression
• interpersonal psychotherapy
• couples therapy
• dynamic interpersonal psychotherapy.

IAPT is encouraging provision outside hospital – in people's homes, GP practices, JobCentres and other community settings.

Further information
A primary care approach to mental health and wellbeing: case study report on Sandwell, NHS Confederation, November 2012.

Hospital services
Psychiatric hospital services have been progressively scaled down over the past 30 years, as many services are now provided in the community. Acute inpatient wards provide care with intensive medical and nursing support for patients in periods of acute illness. Patients usually spend fewer than 90 days on such wards. Psychiatric intensive care units are secure, with staffing levels usually in line with those of ICUs in acute hospitals. Patients are usually detained under the Mental Health Act, but length of stay ranges from a few days to a few weeks.

Child and adolescent mental health services
One in ten children has a clinically significant mental health problem. At any one time, more than a million children will have a diagnosable mental health disorder. Child and adolescent mental health services (CAMHS) cater for those with all types of mental disorder. Services are arranged into four tiers, which should be closely linked:
- tier 1 includes services contributing to mental healthcare of children and young people, but whose primary function is not mental healthcare (for example, schools and GPs)
- tier 2 includes mental health professionals assessing and treating those who do not respond at tier 1
- tier 3 includes teams of mental health professionals providing multi-disciplinary interventions for more complex problems
- tier 4 includes the most severe and complex problems that cannot be dealt with at tier 3, including inpatient and specialist services for conditions such as eating disorders.

NHS and foundation trusts are the principal providers of CAMHS, although local authorities and the independent sector also provide services.

Forensic services
Forensic mental health services deal with mentally ill people who may need a degree of physical security and have shown challenging behaviour beyond the scope of general psychiatric services. Some may be mentally disordered offenders.

Services fall into three categories:

- low-security services tend to be based near general psychiatric wards in
  NHS hospitals, and are for people detained under the Mental Health Act
  who pose a level of risk or challenge so cannot be treated in open settings
- medium-security services often operate regionally and are provided by
  NHS and independent sector organisations; they usually consist of locked
  wards with a greater number and a wider range of staff, and typically
  patients – who may have a history of offending or have been transferred
  from prison or court – remain in treatment between two and five years
- high-security services are provided by the three special hospitals (Ashworth,
  Broadmoor and Rampton), which have much greater levels of security
  and care for people who pose an immediate and serious risk to others.

Care for groups with special needs

Healthcare for people with learning disabilities
There are 985,000 people in England with a learning disability – 2 per cent
of the population – and numbers will increase significantly in the next
15 years, especially among older age groups. But only 177,000 are known
to use learning disability services. People with learning disabilities have
greater health needs than the general population, being more likely to
experience mental illness and more prone to chronic health problems
such as epilepsy, cerebral palsy and other physical disabilities. They are
also 58 times more likely to die before the age of 50. But many have
difficulty accessing healthcare and are less likely to seek routine screening.

When they do access health services they may be subject to 'diagnostic
overshadowing' bias – clinicians' tendency to overlook symptoms of
mental health problems among people with learning disabilities,
attributing them to the disability. Therefore, people with learning
disabilities may need support when using mainstream services, including
longer appointments and help with communication.

The 2001 learning disability white paper, *Valuing people*, was based on four key principles that still apply:

- legal and civil rights – people with learning disabilities have the right to a decent education, to grow up to vote, marry and have a family, and express their opinions, with help and support where necessary
- independence – individuals' needs will differ, but the presumption should be one of independence rather than dependence, with public services providing the support needed to maximise this
- choice – everyone should be able to make choices, including people with severe and profound disabilities, with help and support
- inclusion – people with learning disabilities should be able to do ordinary things, make use of mainstream services and be fully included in the local community.

A follow-up white paper, *Valuing people now*, set out priorities that remain national policy. They include:

- increasing the range of housing options for people with learning disabilities and their families
- ensuring all local authority services and developments for people with learning disabilities and their carers are underpinned by person-centred planning
- increasing employment opportunities.

Following the discovery of systematic abuse of patients by staff at Winterbourne View, an independent hospital in Gloucestershire for people with learning disabilities and challenging behaviour, the Care Quality Commission launched unannounced inspections of 150 services providing care for people with learning disabilities. It found that half failed to meet standards. The Government devised a 60-point programme to improve services, including a pledge that none of the 3,000 people with learning disabilities in long-stay institutions should remain there unless they need to.

Further information

DH Winterbourne View review – concordat: programme of action, DH and partners, December 2012.

Learning disability services inspection programme: national overview, CQC, June 2012.

Valuing people now: a new three-year strategy for people with learning disabilities, HM Government, January 2009.

Valuing people: a new strategy for learning disability for the 21st century, DH, March 2001.

Offender health

People in prison have generally poorer health than the population at large: 71 per cent have two or more mental disorders, and 70 per cent have a concurrent drug and/or alcohol problem; 10 per cent suffer from psychosis, while 80 per cent smoke. The ideal is to provide prisoners with access to the same quality and range of healthcare services as the public receives from the NHS. Schemes to tackle smoking and drug misuse and vaccinate against hepatitis B are common. Prisons have also implemented a care-planning system for prisoners at risk of suicide.

In its role as commissioner of all specialised services, NHS England is now responsible for commissioning healthcare for offenders. It intends to introduce a consistent national approach, coordinated by its four regional teams. As well as covering 120 prisons and young offender institutions, the remit includes:
- 16 secure children's homes
- four secure training centres
- 12 immigration removal centres
- police custody suites
- courts.

Further information

Securing excellence in commissioning for offender health, NHS Commissioning Board, February 2013.

04 Quality and safety

The NHS is committed to providing high-quality care, which means continually striving to improve clinical standards and patient experience, using resources efficiently and ensuring patients' safety. Criteria are set and monitored nationally, with every organisation's performance assessed and made public. Concerns about healthcare-acquired infections and variations in outcomes have brought renewed emphasis on patient safety and effectiveness – reinforced by the findings of the Francis Inquiry into poor care at Mid Staffordshire NHS Foundation Trust.

Ensuring quality

Defining quality
High-quality care comprises three essential dimensions:
• clinical effectiveness – it is based on best evidence about what is clinically effective in improving an individual's health
• safety – it is delivered so as to prevent all avoidable harm and risks to the individual's safety
• patient experience – the individual undergoes as positive an experience of receiving and recovering from care as possible, including being treated according to what they want or need, with compassion, dignity and respect.

Quality is 'systemic' – not a single individual's responsibility but a collective endeavour requiring effort and collaboration at every level of an organisation.

NHS organisations have a statutory duty to ensure the quality of their services, just as they have always had to keep their organisations financially solvent. Indeed, by law they now have to publish 'quality accounts' (see page 75). Other measures designed to foster quality include quality surveillance groups (see page 79), CQUIN (see page 75), adjustments to the tariff system to link increases in payments to specific quality goals (see page 114), registration with the Care Quality Commission (see page 102) and licensing by Monitor (see page 102). In addition, the Government is expanding use of patient-reported outcome measures (see page 78), NICE quality standards (see page 77), national clinical audit and patient surveys. Instead of using targets to measure NHS organisations' performance, they will be judged on the outcomes they achieve (see page 80).

Further information
Quality in the new health system – maintaining and improving quality from April 2013: final report, NQB, January 2013.

National Quality Board

The NQB is intended to provide strategic oversight and leadership in quality across the NHS. Members include the NHS medical director, chief medical and nursing officers and the chairs of the Care Quality Commission, NICE and Monitor, as well as leaders from the third sector, academe, social care and the Royal Colleges.

The board's role is to ensure 'the overall alignment of the systems for managing and improving quality' throughout the NHS. It oversees work to improve quality indicators and advises the Secretary of State on priorities for clinical standards set by NICE.

Quality governance

Monitor (see page 100) defines quality governance as 'the combination of structures and processes at and below board level to lead on trust-wide quality performance'. It includes:

- ensuring required standards are achieved
- investigating and taking action on substandard performance
- planning and driving continuous improvement
- identifying, sharing and ensuring delivery of best practice
- identifying and managing risks to quality of care.

Boards' and governing bodies' responsibilities for quality are to ensure:

- the essential standards of quality and safety (as determined by the CQC's registration requirements – see page 102) are at a minimum being met by every service
- the organisation is striving for continuous quality improvement in every service
- every staff member who has contact with patients, or whose actions directly impact on patient care, is motivated and enabled to deliver effective, safe and person-centred care.

Boards and governing bodies should encourage a culture where services are improved by learning from mistakes: staff, patients and their families should be encouraged to identify areas for improvement and not be afraid to speak out.

Quality governance involves formulating a strategy; ensuring the organisation has the requisite capabilities; fostering an appropriate culture; putting in place the necessary processes and structures and measuring outcomes. Quality governance arrangements should complement, and be fully integrated with, the governance arrangements for other board responsibilities, such as finance governance and research governance.

Further information
Discussion paper 14: Making it better? Assuring high-quality care in the NHS, NHS Confederation, February 2013.
Quality governance in the NHS – a guide for provider boards, NQB, March 2011.

Clinical audit

Clinical audit is an important instrument of quality governance, providing rich data to support service improvement, better information for patients and revalidation of clinicians (see page 106). It 'aims to assess the extent to which care is consistent with best practice and/or achieves expected outcomes'. All healthcare professions undertake clinical audit. With education and research it is one of the medical profession's three core responsibilities, but unlike them has lacked a national strategy and coherent programme – despite participation being mandatory for all doctors since 1989.

The National Advisory Group on Clinical Audit and Enquiries (NAGCAE) is a 'wide and inclusive' forum to enhance the existing programme of national clinical audits and support NHS staff involved in audits in their own organisations. It also seeks to improve connections between national clinical audits regardless of how they are funded, between audit and IT, revalidation and research and development.

NAGCAE also acts as the steering group for the National Clinical Audit and Patients' Outcomes Programme, which commissions national audits, consults those with an interest in audit and develops resources for them. NCAPOP is administered by the Healthcare Quality Improvement Partnership (HQIP), a consortium of the Royal College of Nursing, Academy of Medical Royal Colleges and National Voices.

Further information
Healthcare Quality Improvement Partnership **www.hqip.org.uk**

National service frameworks and strategies

National service frameworks (NSFs) and strategies are evidence-based programmes setting quality standards and specifying services that should be available for a particular condition or care group across the whole NHS. They are intended to eradicate local variations in standards and services, raise standards generally, promote collaboration between organisations and contribute to improving public health. Each identifies key interventions, puts in place a strategy to support implementation and establishes an agreed timescale.

Each NSF was developed with assistance from health professionals, service users and carers, health service managers, partner agencies and other advocates. The DH supported the groups and managed the overall process. They cover:
• cancer
• child health and maternity
• coronary heart disease
• chronic obstructive pulmonary disease
• diabetes
• kidney disease
• long-term conditions
• mental health
• older people
• stroke.

Quality accounts
All providers of NHS care must publish an annual 'quality account' indicating the quality of the care they provide, just as they publish financial accounts. These must be published by June to cover the preceding financial year.

Quality accounts require boards to consider the quality of their services, their priorities for improvement and how they intend to achieve them. Providers are required to include a statement in their quality account which details the national clinical audits and confidential inquiries they have participated in during the year. They are not intended to be a comprehensive assessment of every service, nor to supply patients with information they need to make an informed choice about services, although they are published on the NHS Choices website. Acute and mental health trusts must have their quality accounts externally audited, and include within them opinions from commissioners and key stakeholders such as patient groups.

CQUIN
The Commissioning for Quality and Innovation (CQUIN) payment framework makes part of a provider's income conditional on quality and innovation. It is intended to ensure contracts include quality improvement

plans by allowing commissioners to link a specific proportion of providers' contract income to achieving locally agreed goals. For example, if a commissioner has concerns about stroke services, the provider could undertake to increase the percentage of stroke patients with access to scanning within three hours of admission – a process known to improve outcomes – to an agreed level.

In 2013/14, the amount that can be earned under CQUIN is 2.5 per cent of contract income. All CQUIN schemes are required to include four national goals:
• use the friends and family test (see page 79)
• use the 'NHS safety thermometer' (see page 82)
• improve dementia care
• reduce avoidable death, disability and chronic ill health from venous thromboembolism.

Further information
Commissioning for quality and innovation (CQUIN): 2013/14 guidance,
NHS Commissioning Board, December 2012.

Quality and Outcomes Framework
The QOF is a voluntary incentive scheme to encourage high-quality services in general practice, and was introduced as part of the general medical services contract in 2004. It sets out a range of national standards based on the best available research evidence. The standards are divided into four domains:
• clinical standards linked to the care of patients suffering from chronic disease
• public health and primary prevention indicators, plus additional services, covering cervical screening, child health surveillance, maternity services and contraceptive services
• quality and productivity, including reviews of data
• patient experience, including assessing access to GP appointments measured by the GP patient survey.

A set of indicators – reviewed annually by NICE – has been developed for each domain to describe different aspects of performance. Practices are free to choose the domains they want to focus on and the quality standards to which they aspire. They receive payments against the indicators, which are adjusted according to list size and prevalence of disease. About 15 per cent of practice payments nationally are made through QOF.

Further information
Quality and Outcomes Framework guidance for GMS contract 2013/14, NHS
Commissioning Board/BMA/NHS Employers, March 2013.

NICE quality standards

NICE (see page 101) has developed a library of quality standards to clarify
the clinical evidence and guidance available to clinicians, commissioners
and patients. They reflect clinical best practice, derived from the best
available evidence from NICE guidance and other sources to provide a set
of specific, concise quality statements and associated measures. Evidence
relating to effectiveness and cost-effectiveness, people's experience of
using services, safety issues, equality and cost impact are considered
during the development process. Produced in collaboration with health
and social care professionals, each makes clear what quality care looks
like, to help end variations in care quality: they are reflected in the
commissioning outcomes indicator set (see page 33) and in payment and
incentive mechanisms such as QOF (see opposite) and CQUIN (see page
75). The Government intends the standards will be central to improving
outcomes, acting as the bridge between the outcomes the NHS seeks to
attain and the processes and structures necessary to do so. They are also
being developed for social care.

Indicators for Quality Improvement

NHS clinical teams have access via the Health and Social Care Information
Centre's website to more than 200 indicators generally accepted as effective
measures of high-quality care. They can use these to assess local quality
improvement. The Indicators for Quality Improvement have been selected
with the Royal Colleges, and they are aligned to the five domains in the
NHS Outcomes Framework (see page 80).
www.hscic.gov.uk/iqi

Patient surveys

Listening to patients' views is essential for a patient-centred health service.
To deliver improvements, the NHS has to know what people need and
expect from it, and how well they think the service has responded to their
needs and expectations. The programme of national patient surveys has
three aims:
- to provide feedback for local quality improvement
- to assess users' experience for performance ratings, inspections and
  reviews
- to monitor patients' experience nationally.

The NHS national patient survey programme is the longest established, and one of the largest, patient survey programmes in the world: since 2002, several million patients have taken part. The Care Quality Commission (see page 99) is now responsible for carrying out national survey programmes on a rolling basis. Recent surveys have included 46,000 patients who attended major accident and emergency departments and 15,000 people using community mental health services.

The GP patient survey (see page 46) is sent twice a year, each time reaching 1.36 million patients of GP practices throughout England. It is now in its seventh year, and asks about aspects of accessing care – from making an appointment and experience of reception through to the clinical consultation – as well as other services such as dentistry and out-of-hours provision.

NHS organisations are required to obtain feedback from their own patients about experiences of care. These surveys are intended to:
• track changes in patients' experience, year on year
• provide information for local quality improvement initiatives
• inform each organisation's performance ratings and the performance indicators.

Trusts can seek support in carrying out their surveys from the NHS survey coordination centre, run by Picker Institute Europe on behalf of the CQC, which can also help patients who are taking part in surveys.

Patients may also rate the service they received in hospital or at a GP practice using the NHS Choices website.

Further information
NHS survey co-ordination centre **www.nhssurveys.org**
GP Patient Survey **www.gp-patient.co.uk**

PROMs
Assessing effectiveness of care means understanding success rates from different treatments, including clinical measures such as mortality or survival rates and measures of clinical improvement. But the patient's perspective is just as important. Patient-reported outcome measures (PROMs) are a method for collecting information on the clinical quality of care as reported by patients themselves. Since 2009 all providers of hip replacements, knee replacements, groin hernia surgery and varicose vein surgery must invite patients undergoing one of these procedures – more

friends and family test

The friends and family test (FFT) is intended to be a simple way to identify good and bad performance in NHS-funded care, and encourage staff to make improvements where services do not live up to expectations.

The test asks a standardised question: 'How likely are you to recommend our ward/A&E department to friends and family if they needed similar care or treatment?' Patients use a six-point scale to answer, ranging from 'extremely likely' to 'extremely unlikely'. Scores are calculated by subtracting the proportion of patients who would not recommend the service from those who would be extremely likely to do so.

Initially the test is for all acute providers of adult NHS-funded care covering services for inpatients and patients discharged from A&E departments.

National publication of hospital, trust and ward-level results will begin in July 2013.

Further information

The NHS friends and family test: publication guidance, DH, February 2013.

than 200,000 a year – to complete a pre-operative PROMs questionnaire. Some months after their operation patients are sent a follow-up questionnaire. The comparable data on their quality of life is then used to calculate a numerical value for the improvement to their health.

Quality surveillance groups

Quality surveillance groups (QSGs) will bring together commissioners, regulators and others to share information on quality in order to spot early signs of problems and take action to prevent more serious quality failures. They will be supported by NHS England and operate at two levels: locally, following the pattern of NHS England's 27 area teams, and in NHS England's four regions.

Local QSGs will consider intelligence in detail and take coordinated action to mitigate quality failure.

Regional QSGs will provide an escalation mechanism for local QSGs. They will assimilate risks and concerns from local QSGs, identifying common or recurring issues that would merit a regional or national response.

NHS CONFEDERATION

QSGs are not statutory bodies with formal powers but forums through which different organisations that do have statutory powers can combine to discharge their responsibilities in a more informed and collaborative way.

Further information
How to establish a quality surveillance group – guidance to the new health system, NQB and partners, January 2013.

Assessing performance: the NHS Outcomes Framework
The NHS Outcomes Framework aims to:
- provide an overview of how the NHS performs nationally
- act as a mechanism to hold NHS England to account
- be a catalyst for quality improvement and outcome measurement throughout the NHS.

It is designed to align with the Public Health (see page 41) and Adult Social Care Outcomes Frameworks to achieve the Government's ambitions for the health and social care system.

The framework contains 34 performance indicators within five domains:
- preventing people from dying prematurely
- enhancing quality of life for people with long-term conditions
- helping people recover from episodes of ill health or following injury
- ensuring people have a positive experience of care
- treating and caring for people in a safe environment and protecting them from avoidable harm.

Individual indicators include reducing premature mortality from the four major causes of death: cardiovascular disease, respiratory disease, liver disease and cancer. Reducing deaths in babies and young children is also included, as well as reducing the number of premature deaths in people with learning disabilities and those with serious mental illness. The NHS will also measure whether young people's and children's experience of care has improved.

In addition, the Government has announced its intention to bolster performance assessment by reintroducing a ratings system. The system is likely to comprise a single aggregate rating for every provider, and cover GP practices, hospitals and care homes. The Care Quality Commission will be responsible for publishing the ratings once the system is implemented.

NHS Improving Quality is part of NHS England and its purpose is to support implementation of the NHS Outcomes Framework by designing and commissioning improvement programmes focused on its five domains. As well as looking at best practice from across the NHS and around the world, NHS IQ draws on the experience of predecessor organisations such as the NHS Institute for Innovation and Improvement and the National Cancer Action Team. NHS IQ is working with trusts, CCGs, commissioning support units and strategic clinical networks.

Further information
Our strategic intent, NHS IQ, March 2013.

Further information
Rating providers for quality: a policy worth pursuing?, Nuffield Trust, March 2013.
The NHS Outcomes Framework 2013/14, DH, November 2012.
The NHS Outcomes Framework 2013/14 mind map, NHS Confederation, November 2012.
Improving health and care: the role of the outcomes frameworks, DH, November 2012.

Ensuring patient safety

The NHS's first priority is its patients' safety. No healthcare system can be entirely risk-free but it must do everything possible to minimise unintended harm, whether from healthcare-associated infections or medical accidents. Failure to do so rapidly undermines public confidence in the system.

Over 1 million patient safety incidents in the NHS are reported every year. Of these:
- 69 per cent result in no harm to the patient
- 24 per cent result in low harm
- 6 per cent result in moderate harm
- 0.6 per cent result in death or severe harm.

Patient safety after Francis

Robert Francis QC's public inquiry into the failures in patient care at Mid Staffordshire NHS Foundation Trust between 2005 and 2009 produced 290 recommendations. The inquiry report, published in February 2013, urged the NHS to alter its culture in order to make patient safety a priority. Francis declared: 'Much of what needs to be done does not require additional financial resources, but changes in attitudes, culture, values and behaviour'. He called in particular for more openness, transparency and candour in the NHS.

The Government responded with plans for a wide range of measures, including:
- introduction of a chief inspector of hospitals (see page 100)
- organisations to be bound by a statutory duty of candour to ensure transparency and honesty about mistakes in all organisations overseen by the CQC
- publication of surgery survival rates in ten specialties
- student nurses to spend a year working as healthcare assistants to ensure they have appropriate values and understand their role
- revalidation for nurses, similar to that already introduced for doctors
- DH civil servants to spend time working in frontline healthcare organisations
- a ban on 'gagging clauses' in employment contracts that have prevented staff speaking out about patient safety
- a 'national barring list' to prevent managers guilty of gross misconduct working in healthcare.

Professor Don Berwick is leading a national patient safety advisory group that will draw up proposals for improving patient safety.

Further information
Patients first and foremost: the initial Government response to the report of the Mid Staffordshire NHS Foundation Trust public inquiry, DH, March 2013.
Report of the Mid Staffordshire NHS Foundation Trust public inquiry (the Francis Report), TSO, February 2013.

Measuring safety: NHS safety thermometer
The 'NHS safety thermometer' is a tool for measuring, monitoring and analysing harm caused to patients and the proportion of care that is 'harm free'. Frontline healthcare professionals use it to take a snapshot once a month to measure harm from four common patient safety problems:
- pressure ulcers

Central Alerting System

The web-based Central Alerting System (CAS) distributes all patient safety alerts and related guidance to the NHS and other health and social care providers. These include emergency alerts, drug alerts, 'Dear Doctor' letters and medical device alerts issued on behalf of the Medicines and Healthcare Products Regulatory Agency and the DH. The public can access CAS, although part of the site is open only to registered NHS users.
www.cas.dh.gov.uk

- falls in care
- urinary infection in patients with a catheter
- treatment for venous thromboembolism.

It can be used for acute care, community hospitals, district nursing caseloads and nursing homes. The thermometer takes only a minimum set of data to signal where individuals, teams and organisations might need to focus more detailed measurement, training and improvement: in effect it highlights abnormal readings and measures changes. It has been designed to measure local improvement over time and not to compare organisations, as differences in patient mix and data collection methods can invalidate such comparisons. For example, trusts with a high percentage of older patients or specialist services are likely to show more harm.

Each month the Health and Social Care Information Centre publishes a national NHS safety thermometer containing data submitted by care providers in the previous month. For example, in September 2012 it contained an aggregate dataset of 706,927 patients submitted by 520 providers of NHS-funded care; 91.3 per cent of patients were found to have received 'harm-free' care.

CQUIN (see page 75) provides an incentive for organisations to use the safety thermometer.

Further information
Delivering the NHS safety thermometer CQUIN 2013/14, NHS Harm Free Care, December 2012.
http://harmfreecare.org/

'Never events' are serious and largely preventable patient safety incidents that can cut life short or result in serious impairment. They should never be allowed to happen in a high-quality service. A list was first drawn up for the NHS in 2009 covering eight never events, including wrong-site surgery, instruments left inside the patient after surgery, inpatient suicide while on one-to-one observation, in-hospital maternal death from post-partum haemorrhage after elective caesarean, and transferred prisoners absconding from medium- or high-secure mental health services.

The list has now been extended to 25 and includes severe scalding, transfusing the wrong type of blood and misidentifying patients by failing to use the standard wristband.

Payment from commissioners may be withheld where never events occur. In 2011/12, there were 326 never events reported, most of them related to surgery.

Further information
The 'never events' list 2012/13, DH, January 2012.

Combating healthcare-associated infections

HCAIs are infections acquired in hospitals or as a result of healthcare interventions. They are caused by a wide variety of micro-organisms, often by bacteria that normally live harmlessly in or on the body. While HCAIs are most likely to be acquired during treatment in acute hospitals, like other bacterial infections they are fairly prevalent in the community and can occur in other care settings. They can have severe consequences for patients as well as costs for the NHS. An HCAI lengthens a patient's stay in hospital and adds to costs.

HCAIs are a worldwide problem. Since the mid-1980s, prevalence in hospitals worldwide has been 5 to 10 per cent; in England it was recorded at 8.2 per cent by 2004. The NHS has had a particular problem with MRSA and C. *difficile*, but a wide range of measures drastically reduced infection rates. In 2012/13 the NHS was asked to reduce MRSA infections by a further 29 per cent and C. *difficile* by 17 per cent.

05 Accountability and regulation

NHS organisations must demonstrate strategic and operational accountability: they must have a clear and well-evidenced long-term plan, and show transparency in their day-to-day decisions. They are accountable to local people who are consumers of their services and to taxpayers who fund the NHS: therefore, they have a duty to maintain the highest standards of quality and safety, as well as to balance the books and provide value for money.

The Government summarised the purpose of its 2013 NHS reorganisation as improving accountability: 'Our aim is to put patients, carers and local communities at the heart of the NHS, shifting decision-making as close as possible to individual patients and carers by devolving power to professionals and providers and liberating them from top-down control.'

Clinical commissioning groups are accountable outwards to their local communities and upwards to NHS England, which in turn is accountable through the Secretary of State to Parliament and the electorate. Foundation trusts are also accountable to their local communities, to Monitor and to Parliament.

NHS organisations are immediately accountable to independently appointed boards, and they have a duty to involve and consult patients and the public. They can also be called to account by their local authority, in particular through the health and wellbeing board. They must also answer to a variety of national regulators and inspectorates. The healthcare professions too are subject to their own regulatory bodies, which set standards and police them.

The role of boards and governing bodies

Duties and responsibilities
In NHS provider organisations, boards take corporate responsibility for their organisation's strategies and actions. With current policy emphasis on decentralisation, local leadership and autonomy, their role is more important than ever.

Boards consist of executives (including the chief executive and finance director) and non-executives plus a chair. The chair and non-executives are lay people drawn from the local community.

A board's role is:
- formulating the organisation's strategy
- holding the organisation to account for achieving the strategy and ensuring that systems of control are robust and reliable
- shaping a positive culture for the board and the organisation.

An effective board:
- is informed by the external context in which it operates
- is informed by and shapes information about the organisation's performance, as well as local people's needs and the market
- builds a healthy dialogue with patients, public and staff, and feels accountable to all of them.

Legally, there is no distinction between the board duties of executive and non-executive directors: they both share responsibility for the organisation's direction and control. The board is expected to bring about change by making best use of all its resources – financial, staffing, physical infrastructure and knowledge – and working with staff and partner organisations to meet the public's and patients' expectations. As leaders, board members are expected to understand opportunities for improving services and motivate others to bring them about.

Boards make plans to achieve the Government's objectives for healthcare, guided by long-term strategy and shorter-term aims such as the NHS Outcomes Framework (see page 80). Boards have increasing scope to pace their plans to reflect local circumstances, and have a large say over how to achieve them – in theory at least. All boards sign off an annual business plan setting out the year's objectives, and it is the whole board's function to ensure progress.

NHS boards are obliged to ensure their organisations have an ethos and culture of public service that reflects and respects public expectation. The need for public accountability means boards must conduct business in an open and transparent way that commands public confidence. Their meetings are usually open to the public, and should be understandable to the public.

Boards and governing bodies have a crucial role to play in bringing about cultural change in the NHS following the Francis Report (see page 82). As part of the Government's response to the report, it is developing a 'barring mechanism' designed to prevent 'unsuitable board-level executives and non-executives from moving to new senior positions elsewhere in the system'. It is also considering 'additional legal sanctions at corporate level' for organisations found to be massaging figures or concealing the truth about their performance.

Meanwhile, Monitor, the Care Quality Commission and the NHS Trust Development Authority are developing a 'fit and proper person test' for board-level directors, which will cover basic issues such as bankruptcy and criminal convictions.

Further information
Leadership in a matrix: a personal view from Ciarán Devane, NHS Confederation, November 2012.
The healthy NHS board: principles for good governance, National Leadership Centre, February 2010.

The chair
The chair's role is to:
- ensure the board develops a vision, strategies and clear objectives to deliver organisational purpose
- hold the chief executive to account for achieving the strategy
- ensure board committees that support accountability are properly constituted
- provide visible leadership in developing a positive culture for the organisation, and ensure this is reflected and modelled in their own and the board's behaviour and decision-making
- lead and support a constructive dynamic within the board, enabling contributions from all directors
- provide a safe point of access to the board for whistle-blowers
- ensure all board members are well briefed on the organisation's external context
- ensure requirements for accurate, timely and clear information to the board directors (and for foundation trusts, governors) are clear
- play a key role as an ambassador and build strong partnerships with patients and public; for foundation trusts, members and governors; clinicians and staff; key institutional stakeholders and regulators.

In general, a strong correlation exists between the quality of the chair's and chief executive's leadership and the organisation's success. Where an organisation is not delivering, questions can legitimately be asked about the quality of the board leadership.

Standards for members of boards and CCG governing bodies

Anticipating the Francis Report (see page 82), the Professional Standards Authority for Health and Social Care (see page 104) produced a set of standards so that board members and those on CCG governing bodies could better understand 'both the extent and limitations of their personal responsibilities'. They emphasise that respect, compassion and care for patients should be at the centre of leadership and good governance.

The standards were produced after consultation with patients, the public, the NHS and professional organisations. They bring together the essential skills that are expected of all executive and non-executive directors in the NHS in England, and cover personal behaviour, technical competence and business practices. They are based on seven core values:
- responsibility
- honesty
- openness
- respect
- professionalism
- leadership
- integrity.

Further information

Standards for members of NHS boards and clinical commissioning group governing bodies in England, Professional Standards Authority, November 2012.
www.professionalstandards.org.uk

Non-executive directors

Non-executive directors should:
- bring independence, external skills and perspectives to strategy development
- hold executives to account for achieving the strategy
- offer purposeful, constructive scrutiny and challenge
- chair or participate as members of key committees that support accountability
- actively support and promote a positive culture for the organisation and reflect this in their own behaviour
- provide a safe point of access to the board for whistle-blowers
- satisfy themselves of the integrity of financial and quality intelligence
- ensure the board acts in the best interests of the public
- ensure a senior independent director is available to members (and in foundation trusts, governors) if there are unresolved concerns.

Further information

Briefing 260: The non-executive directors' guide to hospital data – part one: activity, pathways and datasets, NHS Confederation, March 2013.

The chief executive

The chief executive is responsible for ensuring the board is empowered to govern the organisation and its objectives are accomplished through effective and properly controlled executive action. A chief executive's main responsibilities are:

- leading strategy development
- leading the organisation in achieving the strategy
- establishing effective performance management arrangements and controls
- acting as the organisation's accountable officer
- providing visible leadership in developing a positive culture for the organisation, and ensuring this is reflected in their own and the executive's behaviour and decision-making
- ensuring all board members are well briefed on the organisation's external context
- ensuring provision of accurate, timely and clear information to board directors (and in foundation trusts, governors)
- playing a key role as an ambassador and building strong partnerships with patients and public; for foundation trusts, members and governors; clinicians and staff; key institutional stakeholders and regulators.

Board committees

NHS boards may delegate some of their powers to formally constituted committees. Some are set up to advise the board on a permanent basis, such as the:

- audit committee
- remuneration and terms of service committee
- clinical governance committee
- risk management committee.

Foundation trust boards

Foundation trusts have distinctive governance arrangements. Staff, patients and local people are eligible to become 'members' of the trust. Membership entitles them to vote at elections for the council of governors and to stand for election to it.

The council of governors includes those elected by the trust members and staff, as well as people appointed by local authorities. Representatives

NHS Leadership Academy

The NHS Leadership Academy is the health service's in-house centre for leadership development. It brings together in one body for the first time all national activity supporting leadership development in health and NHS-funded services. The Academy aims to 'professionalise' leadership, raising the profile, performance and impact of leaders in the NHS. It intends that its programmes will create a cadre of leaders at every level and from every professional background equipped to head high-performing organisations. Its 'leadership framework' is a toolkit which sets out a consistent standardised approach to leadership development. The Academy also runs the graduate management training scheme and the top leaders programme.
www.leadershipacademy.nhs.uk

elected by patients and the public must be in the majority, while at least three must be elected by staff. The council of governors' role is to advise the board of directors on its forward plans. It also has the power to remove the chief executive. Governors numbered 4,800 by the end of 2012.

Each foundation trust has a board of directors made up of non-executives appointed by the governors and executive directors appointed by the non-executives. This board is responsible for managing the foundation trust, including its day-to-day operation and forward business plan.

Board of directors' meetings concern the trust's operational business, with council of governors' meetings focusing more on members' needs and ensuring local communities can contribute to decision-making. Since the Health and Social Care Act 2012, foundation trusts must hold their board meetings in public.

The Act conferred a range of new powers and duties on governors, some yet to come into force. For example, they must decide whether the trust's private patient work would significantly interfere with the trust's principal purpose. They must now also hold the non-executive directors to account for their performance, and approve any 'significant transactions'.

Further information

Your statutory duties: a draft reference guide for NHS foundation trust governors, Monitor, December 2012.
Director–governor interaction in NHS foundation trusts: a best practice guide for boards of directors, Monitor/PA Consulting Group, June 2012.

CCGs' governing bodies

Every clinical commissioning group must have a governing body with decision-making powers. By law they must include:

- an accountable officer, who may be an employee or member of the CCG
- a chair, who may be any member of the governing body
- a chief finance officer
- a healthcare professional acting on behalf of member practices
- a lay member with responsibility for governance
- a lay member with responsibility for championing patient and public involvement
- a clinical member who is a secondary care doctor
- a clinical member who is a registered nurse.

If the chair is a GP or other healthcare professional, the deputy chair must be a lay member. CCGs are otherwise free to choose the number of members on their governing body and the background from which they come.

Further information

Clinical commissioning group governing body members: role outlines, attributes and skills, NHS Commissioning Board, April 2012.

Engaging patients and the public

Patient and public engagement is the active participation of patients, carers, community representatives, community groups and the public in how services are planned, delivered and evaluated. It is broader and deeper than traditional consultation. It involves the ongoing process of developing and sustaining constructive relationships, building strong, active partnerships and holding a meaningful dialogue with stakeholders.

Engaging with patients and the public can happen at two levels: individuals have a say in decisions about their own care and treatment, while collectively, communities influence decisions about commissioning and delivery of services.

Effective patient engagement means involving patient cohorts in helping to get the service right for them. It is also about engaging the public in decisions about the commissioning, planning, design and reconfiguration of health services, either proactively as design partners, or reactively, through consultation. Effective engagement leads to improvements in health services.

'The NHS belongs to the people...' The NHS Constitution, which applies only to the health service in England, comprises:

- seven key principles that govern how the NHS operates, such as providing a comprehensive service and aspiring to put patients 'at the heart of everything it does'
- six values, including respect and dignity, commitment to quality and compassion
- legal rights and pledges to patients and the public about matters such as access, quality, respect, choice and complaints
- responsibilities that patients and public owe the NHS, such as keeping appointments and treating staff with respect
- staff's legal rights and pledges to them concerning issues such as working environment, fair pay, representation and equal treatment
- staff's legal duties and responsibilities, including patient confidentiality and professional accountability.

The Health Act 2009 placed a duty on all NHS organisations, private and third sector providers in England to take account of the Constitution. By law the Government must renew the Constitution every ten years, so that changes cannot take place without debate.

After the 2010 election, the current Government pledged: 'We will uphold the NHS Constitution', although it has made changes. In 2012 several measures highlighting the importance of whistle-blowing were added. Further changes in 2013 concerned the duty of candour, feedback, patient involvement, complaints, end-of-life care, dignity, respect and compassion. A public health supplement was also published.

Further information

The NHS Constitution for England, NHS, March 2013.
The handbook to the NHS Constitution for England, DH, March 2013.
Public health supplement to the NHS Constitution, DH/LGA/PHE, March 2013.

Since 2000 the health service has had an explicit duty to ensure patients and the public have a real say in how services are planned and developed. Further legislation in 2006 and 2007 strengthened the duty to involve and consult service users or their representatives.

The NHS Constitution establishes as an underlying principle that the health service will involve individual patients and the wider community, and be accountable to the public, communities and patients. It includes specific rights for patients to be involved in discussions and decisions about their healthcare, in planning healthcare services and in decisions about proposed changes and how services are run. The NHS also pledges to provide the information needed to enable this to happen.

The Health and Social Care Act 2012 continues this process. The Government's *Liberating the NHS* white paper in 2010 declared that the slogan 'no decision about me without me' should come to epitomise an NHS where patients are involved fully in their own care, with decisions made in partnership with clinicians rather than by clinicians alone.

Health and wellbeing boards (see page 19) have a duty to involve users and the public, while CCGs must state in their annual commissioning plans how they intend to involve patients and the public in commissioning decisions. CCGs and NHS England have to involve the public in any changes that affect patient services, not just those with a 'significant' impact. NHS England assesses how effectively CCGs have discharged their duty to involve patients and the public as part of their annual assessment.

Further information
The patient experience book: a collection of the NHS Institute for Innovation and Improvement's guidance and support, NHS Institute, March 2013.
Feeling better? Improving patient experience in hospital, NHS Confederation, January 2011.
Liberating the NHS: local democratic legitimacy in health, DH, July 2010.

HealthWatch
HealthWatch is designed to be the new 'consumer champion' for health and adult social care. It exists in two distinct forms: local HealthWatch and, at national level, HealthWatch England.

Local HealthWatch evolved from the existing 150 local involvement networks (LINks), the main vehicles for involving patients and the public in the NHS since 2008, but has additional functions and powers to hold to account local services. The aim is to give citizens and communities a stronger voice to influence and challenge how health and social care services are provided within their locality. Each is an independent organisation, able to employ its own staff and volunteers. The 152 local HealthWatch organisations are not accountable to HealthWatch England but to their local authorities.

At local level, HealthWatch:
- ensures patients' and carers' views influence commissioning, through a seat on the health and wellbeing board
- provides advocacy and support to patients making a complaint
- feeds intelligence to HealthWatch England, alerting it to concerns about specific providers.

Commissioners and providers have a duty to pay due regard to findings from local HealthWatch organisations. Local HealthWatch membership must be representative of local people and different users of services, including carers.

HealthWatch England is a national body that enables the collective views of NHS and social care users to influence national policy. It is a statutory committee of the Care Quality Commission and funded through it, with a chair who is a CQC non-executive director. It:
- provides leadership, advice and support to local HealthWatch
- provides advice to the Secretary of State, NHS England, Monitor and the English local authorities – to which they must pay regard
- proposes CQC investigations of poor services.

Further information
Local HealthWatch: a strong voice for people – the policy explained, DH, March 2012.
www.healthwatch.co.uk

Patient advice and liaison services
Every hospital should have a patient advice and liaison service (PALS) providing on-the-spot help and information about health services. PALS aim to:
- provide information to patients, carers and their families about local health services and put people in contact with local support groups
- tell people about the complaints procedure and independent complaints advocacy support
- act as an early-warning system by monitoring trends, highlighting gaps in service and making reports for action to managers.

The National PALS Network aims to promote PALS and support the professional development of PALS staff, as well as acting as a national voice for the service.

Further information
National PALS Network www.networks.nhs.uk/nhs-networks/national-pals-network

Complaints

Reforming complaints procedures
Since 2009, a single complaints system has existed for all health and local authority adult social care services in England. These unified arrangements aim to:
- resolve complaints locally in a more personal and flexible way
- ensure early and effective resolution and robust handling of all cases, not just the more complex
- make sure people with complaints have access to effective support, particularly those who find it difficult to make their views heard
- give people the option of going direct to the commissioner with a complaint about their GP, NHS dentist or pharmacist instead of complaining directly to the practice
- give people the option of going direct to their local authority where their care has been arranged by the local authority
- ensure organisations improve services by routinely learning from people's experiences.

The range of measures available locally to resolve complaints include:
- robust risk assessment to quickly deal with serious complaints, such as those involving abuse or unsafe practice
- a plan, agreed by the complainant, outlining how the complaint is going to be tackled, who will be involved and their roles, timescales and how the complainant will be kept informed of progress
- involvement of the most senior managers or clinicians at an early stage where appropriate
- early face-to-face meetings between everyone concerned to make sure the circumstances giving rise to the complaint are clearly understood
- independent mediators when the relationship between the complainant and the NHS body has broken down
- people independent of the service provider, commissioning organisation or the locality to investigate where complaints cannot be resolved satisfactorily or complex issues are involved
- specialist advocates to help people with complex needs voice their complaint effectively and understand the organisation's response
- clear, effective leadership from the most senior managers to ensure complaints arrangements meet people's needs and services are improved as a result.

Local organisations must make every effort to resolve the complaint, but if complainants are dissatisfied with the local response they may go directly to the Ombudsman.

In 2011/12, the NHS received 162,129 complaints, an 8.3 per cent increase on the previous year. The Government ordered a review of how the NHS handles complaints, led by Ann Clwyd MP, following the Francis Report. It is due to conclude in summer 2013.

The Ombudsman
The office of the Parliamentary and Health Service Ombudsman undertakes independent investigations into complaints about the NHS in England, as well as government departments and other public bodies. It is completely independent of the NHS and Government. In the NHS, the Ombudsman investigates complaints that a hardship or injustice has been caused by its failure to provide a service, by a failure in service or by maladministration. The Ombudsman looks into complaints against private health providers only if the treatment was funded by the NHS.

Complainants can only take their cases to the Ombudsman if they fail to achieve a resolution with the organisation or practitioner they are complaining against – for example, because of delays in dealing with a complaint locally or failure to get a satisfactory answer. The Ombudsman can consider complaints from a patient; a close member of the family, partner or representative, if the patient is unable to act for themselves; or from someone who has suffered injustice or hardship as a result of the actions of the NHS. A complaint will normally only be considered within a year of the events which gave rise to it, and only if the Ombudsman believes the NHS has not acted properly or has provided a poor service.

The Ombudsman publishes detailed reports of investigations, which identify common themes in complaints. The reports are intended to be used as training tools to improve services, and chief executives are asked to ensure all clinical directors and complaints managers are aware of them. They are also considered by the House of Commons public administration committee, which is currently inquiring into NHS complaints handling.
www.ombudsman.org.uk

NHSLA, set up in 1995, handles negligence claims against NHS bodies in England, and operates a risk management programme to help raise standards and reduce incidents leading to claims. It also monitors human rights case law and coordinates equal-pay claims on the NHS's behalf.

In 2011/12 NHSLA received 9,143 claims for clinical negligence and paid out £1.2 billion in damages and costs, a 67 per cent increase in five years. At March 2012 it had 22,512 live claims. Fewer than 50 clinical negligence cases a year are contested in court, and 96 per cent of the NHSLA's cases are settled out of court. Claims are settled on average in a year and three months. Of all clinical claims handled since 2002:
• 35.3 per cent were abandoned by the claimant
• 45.5 per cent were settled out of court
• 2.6 per cent were settled in court
• 15.4 per cent are outstanding.

The National Clinical Assessment Service, which helps resolve concerns about the professional practice of doctors, dentists and pharmacists, became part of NHSLA in 2013.
www.nhsla.com

Reforming clinical negligence procedures

Although the NHS provides high-quality healthcare for millions of people every year, occasionally patients do not receive the treatment they should, or mistakes are made. In the UK and other developed countries, about 10 per cent of hospital admissions may result in some kind of adverse event, and a third of these patients will suffer severe illness or die. In NHS primary care, research suggests about 600 errors a day occur, mainly in diagnosis and treatment, of which a fifth will cause harm.

Anyone who suffers harm as a result of treatment must receive an apology, a clear explanation of what went wrong, proper treatment and care and, where appropriate, financial compensation. The NHS must ensure it learns from such experiences.

But legal proceedings for medical injury are slow, complex and costly. They divert clinical staff from providing care, and can damage morale as well as public confidence. The system encourages defensiveness and secrecy, which hampers the NHS from learning and improvement.

The NHS Redress Act 2006 provided an alternative to litigation for less severe and less costly cases, aimed at shifting emphasis from attributing blame towards preventing harm, reducing risks and learning from mistakes, while avoiding the courts altogether. However, ministers decided against implementing the scheme.

The number and cost of clinical negligence claims against the NHS have surged in recent years. Research suggests costs are being driven by the use of 'no win, no fee' lawyers, and often claimants' costs are disproportionate to the damages paid, particularly in low-value claims. Changes to the rules on lawyers' conditional fees, which came into effect in April 2013, may help stem rising costs.

Regulation and inspection

NHS organisations and the healthcare professions are all subject to stringent regulation, audit and inspection to ensure they maintain high service standards and provide value for money.

The regulators

Many national bodies are responsible for regulating, auditing and inspecting various aspects of NHS services – some long-established, others more recent. Regulation covers numerous areas but is essentially a way of preventing conditions that may adversely affect patients' interests. It has helped mitigate against limited access to services, high prices, perverse incentives and lack of information, as well as ensuring safety and quality.

The following are among the major national bodies regulating and inspecting the NHS:

Care Quality Commission

Operating since 2009, the CQC regulates the quality and safety of health and adult social care services, whether provided by the NHS, local authorities, private companies or voluntary organisations. Its functions are:
- registering health and adult social care providers to ensure they meet essential common safety and quality standards
- monitoring and inspecting all health and adult social care, including how the Mental Health Act is working
- using enforcement powers, such as fines, public warnings or closures, if standards are not met
- reporting the outcomes of its work to the public and professionals.

chief inspector of hospitals

As part of the Government's response to the Francis Report, the Care Quality Commission is to appoint a chief inspector of hospitals, who will assess every NHS hospital's performance, drawing on the views of commissioners, local patients and the public. The chief inspector will be helped by the 'expert judgements of inspectors who have walked the wards, spoken to patients and staff, and looked the board in the eye', according to the Government.

'Just as OFSTED acts as a credible, respected and independent arbiter of the best and the worst in our schools, the chief inspector will become the nation's whistle-blower – naming poor care without fear or favour from politicians, institutional vested interests or through loyalty to the system rather than the patients that it serves', the Government says. It is also to consider appointing a chief inspector of primary care.

Since 2010, health and adult social care providers must register with the CQC in order to provide services. The CQC hosts HealthWatch England (see page 94).

After criticism from the Commons public accounts committee and others that the CQC was ineffective, it increased the number of compliance inspectors and improved their training. All inspections are now unannounced. Once the chief inspector of hospitals is established (see box), the CQC will take the lead in quality surveillance groups (see page 79) in assessing quality problems; Monitor and the NHS Trust Development Authority will lead on overseeing action to address them.

Further information

The Care Quality Commission: regulating the quality and safety of health and adult social care – seventy-eighth report of session 2010–12, House of Commons public accounts committee, March 2012.
www.cqc.org.uk

Monitor

Established in 2004, Monitor's original function was authorising and regulating NHS foundation trusts. It is now the sector regulator for healthcare, whose main duty is 'to protect and promote the interests of patients' by promoting efficient, effective and economic provision of services.

In addition to assessing NHS trusts applying for foundation trust status, Monitor's other roles are:
- licensing providers of NHS care – see page 102
- from 2014/15, setting prices for NHS-funded care in partnership with NHS England, with the results published in the national tariff
- enabling integrated care where it improves service quality, access or efficiency
- safeguarding choice and preventing anti-competitive behaviour but not promoting competition for its own sake
- ensuring the continuity of services, monitoring providers' finances and intervening if patients' access to services could be in danger.

Further information
An introduction to Monitor's role, Monitor, April 2013.
www.monitor-nhsft.gov.uk

National Institute for Health and Care Excellence (NICE)
NICE was set up in 1999 to reduce variation in the availability and quality of NHS treatments and care – the so-called 'postcode lottery'. Its evidence-based guidance helps resolve uncertainty about which medicines, treatments, procedures and devices represent the best quality care and which offer the best value for money. It also produces public health guidance, recommending best ways to encourage healthy living, promote wellbeing and prevent disease.

All its guidance and quality standards are developed by an independent committee of experts including clinicians, patients, carers and health economists. NICE's 30-strong citizens council provides it with advice that reflects the public's perspective on what are often challenging social and moral issues raised by NICE guidance. Under the NHS Constitution, patients have a right to treatments NICE has recommended.

The NHS Outcomes Framework (see page 80) is linked to NICE's quality standards (see page 77), while under the Health and Social Care Act 2012, NICE's remit was extended to produce quality standards for social care. NICE will take responsibility for assessing the full value of medicines when new pricing arrangements are introduced in 2014.
www.nice.org.uk

registration and licensing

The Care Quality Commission and Monitor operate a single, integrated process of registration and licensing for all health and social care services in England.

Since 2010 all providers of certain health and social care services have had to register with the CQC and demonstrate that they meet a single set of essential standards for quality and safety of care. Without registering, it is illegal for organisations to provide certain services. There are 16 standards grouped into five areas:
• treating people with respect and involving them in their care
• provision of care, treatment and support that meets people's needs
• caring for people safely and protecting them from harm
• suitability of staffing
• suitability of management.

To maintain their registration, providers must demonstrate a continuing ability to meet all the standards.

All providers of NHS care will soon require a licence from Monitor unless they are exempt under regulations: foundation trusts have needed a licence since April 2013; all others will do so from April 2014. It will be used to:
• support commissioners to secure continuity of NHS services
• enforce prices for NHS services
• address providers' anti-competitive behaviour that is against patients' interests
• enable integrated care
• oversee the governance of NHS foundation trusts.

Further information

Protecting and promoting patients' interests – licensing providers of NHS services: summary of responses to the consultation, DH, March 2013.

The new NHS provider licence, Monitor, February 2013.

Briefing 257: All systems go – testing the new licensing system for providers of NHS-funded care, NHS Confederation, December 2012.

Essential standards of quality and safety: guidance about compliance, CQC, March 2010.

National Audit Office

Headed by the Comptroller and Auditor General, the NAO's role is to report direct to Parliament on how public bodies have spent central government money, conducting financial audits and assessing value for money. It works closely with the Commons public accounts committee (see page 14).
www.nao.org.uk

Local authorities

Since April 2013 the health scrutiny functions formerly invested in a local authority's health overview and scrutiny committee are now invested in the local authority itself. The new arrangements include:

- extending scrutiny to all providers of NHS care, whether a hospital, charity or independent provider
- requiring organisations proposing substantial service changes, and the local authorities scrutinising those proposals, to publish clear timescales for decision-making
- requiring local authorities to take account of the financial sustainability of services when considering whether to make any changes
- seeking NHS England's help in liaising with local authorities and commissioners to secure local agreement on some service reconfigurations.

The Centre for Public Scrutiny has helped to foster local authorities' role in scrutinising health services.

Further information

Health and Social Care Act 2012: briefing for overview and scrutiny members and officers, CfPS, June 2012.
Centre for Public Scrutiny: **www.cfps.org.uk**

Professional regulation

NHS patients need to know that the staff who care for them are well-trained and competent. Professional self-regulation has been a cornerstone of the NHS since it began, yet events in the last 15 years – such as the Bristol Inquiry into the deaths of child heart patients (1998–2001), the Alder Hey cases in which organs from dead children were retained without their families' knowledge (2001), Dr Harold Shipman's conviction for multiple murders (2000) and failures in patient care at Mid Staffordshire NHS Foundation trust (2005–09) – highlighted the need for reform.

Professional Standards Authority for Health and Social Care

The Professional Standards Authority for Health and Social Care (formerly the Council for Healthcare Regulatory Excellence) is a statutory body responsible to Parliament and independent of the Department of Health. It covers all the UK, promoting best practice and consistency in professional self-regulation in nine bodies that cover 1.2 million health professionals in 31 different health professions:

- General Medical Council
- General Dental Council
- General Optical Council
- General Osteopathic Council
- General Chiropractic Council
- Health and Care Professions Council
- Nursing and Midwifery Council
- General Pharmaceutical Council
- Pharmaceutical Society of Northern Ireland.

Unlike the CHRE, the Professional Standards Authority is funded through a levy on the professional regulators and its remit extends to social work in England.
www.professionalstandards.org.uk

Professional regulation covers education, registration, training, continuing professional development and revalidation. It includes setting standards for deciding who should enter and remain members of a profession and determining their fitness to practise. Its underpinning principles are:

- clarity about standards
- maintaining public confidence
- transparency in tackling fitness to practise
- responsiveness to and protection of patients.

Professional regulation issues and initiatives are usually UK-wide.

Professional regulatory bodies

During the past decade and especially since reforms in 2008, regulatory bodies have become smaller, with many more public and patient representatives. They have striven for faster, more transparent procedures and more meaningful accountability to the public and the health service. They have also developed common systems across the professions and agreed standards that put patients' interests first. Professional regulatory bodies must be open and make improvements based on feedback from patients, their representatives and the public. They must deal with complaints quickly, thoroughly, objectively and in a way that is responsive to the complainant while treating fairly the health professional complained against.

Updated regulatory bodies have been introduced for medicine, nursing, midwifery and health visiting, the allied health professions and pharmacy:

- **The General Medical Council** is the regulatory body for doctors. Since 2009, all doctors must be both registered and hold a licence to practise; they must renew their licence periodically through revalidation (see page 106). In 2011 the GMC received 8,781 inquiries about doctors' fitness to practise, of which 56 per cent were closed with no action taken.
www.gmc-uk.org
- **The Nursing and Midwifery Council** replaced the UK Central Council in 2002 as the body responsible for governing nurses, midwives and health visitors.
www.nmc-uk.org
- **The Health and Care Professions Council** is responsible for the professions previously regulated by the Council for Professions Supplementary to Medicine, and includes groups of healthcare professionals not previously covered by formal statutory regulation.
www.hpc-uk.org
- **The General Dental Council** and **General Optical Council** regulate the dental and optometry professions.
GDC www.gdc-uk.org
GOC www.optical.org
- **The General Pharmaceutical Council** replaced the Royal Pharmaceutical Society of Great Britain in 2010 as the regulator for pharmacists and pharmacy technicians.
www.pharmacyregulation.org

Professional regulators are undergoing increased scrutiny. Since 2012 the Law Commission has been reviewing the legislation on regulating healthcare professionals with the aim of simplifying the law and establishing a streamlined, transparent and responsive system of regulation. The former Council for Healthcare Regulatory Excellence criticised the Nursing and Midwifery Council (NMC) in a strategic review of the organisation in 2012, highlighting problems 'at every level' and noting it had failed to become 'the modern, effective and efficient regulator that the public, nurses and midwives need and deserve'.

Medical revalidation is the process by which doctors have to demonstrate to the GMC, normally every five years, that they are fit to practise and are up to date with the latest techniques, technologies and research. It requires a doctor to tackle any concerns about skills, such as communication and maintaining trust with patients. It applies to all doctors in the UK, including locums and those working in the private sector – more than 218,000 in total. The DH claims they are the first in the world to have regular assessments of their training and expertise.

Revalidation began in December 2012, but has a long history, being first proposed by the GMC in 2000. The Shipman Inquiry in 2004 identified it as a key factor in improving patient safety. It represents a new way of regulating the medical profession that focuses on doctors' efforts to maintain and improve their practice.

It is based on a local evaluation of doctors' performance through an annual appraisal, at which a portfolio of supporting information is used as a basis for discussion. Evidence from appraisals must include examples of quality improvement, any significant events and feedback from colleagues and patients. Information from the appraisal is provided to a 'responsible officer' – for example, a trust medical director – who recommends to the GMC whether to revalidate the doctor.

Revalidation is forecast to cost the NHS £970 million over the next ten years but produce net savings of £78.5 million by 2022 once the benefits of reduced harm to patients, fewer suspended doctors and a fall in litigation costs are taken into account.

The Government now intends to work with the NMC to produce a 'proportionate and affordable' system of revalidation for nurses.

Further information

Medical revalidation – costs and benefits: analysis of the costs and benefits of medical revalidation in England, DH, November 2012.
NHS Revalidation Support Team **www.revalidationsupport.nhs.uk**

The Francis Report (see page 82) urged the GMC and NMC to act more quickly on concerns, share information more proactively with other regulators and put greater emphasis on protecting patients and the public. In response, the Government has pledged to overhaul current complex legislation to enable 'faster and more proactive action on individual professional failings'.

Further information
Strategic review of the Nursing and Midwifery Council: final report, CHRE, July 2012.
Regulation of health care professionals; regulation of social care professionals in England, Law Commission, March 2012.

Regulating managers

NHS managers carry great responsibility for ensuring patient safety and deploying public money; failures of management can result in death or harm to patients. Therefore it is essential that mechanisms exist to guarantee the calibre of NHS managers. In the light of the Mid Staffordshire Inquiry and other cases of management failure, the public has had particular concerns about unsuitable board-level directors and non-executives moving to new positions elsewhere in the system.

Following the Francis Report, the Government announced plans to develop a 'barring mechanism', which would ensure that 'individuals whose conduct or competence makes them unsuitable for these vital roles are prevented from securing them'. This will need to be fair, independent and effective, enhancing professional esteem for the majority of senior leaders while not discouraging capable and experienced people from serving in both executive and non-executive roles.

Proposals will be published after consultation, which will also consider whether the scheme should be extended beyond board level to other managers.

06 Financing the NHS

While the NHS has embraced diversity in the provision of its services, its funding continues to draw overwhelmingly on a single source – taxation – although it does raise a certain amount from charges. However, the way money flows through the system has been drastically reformed with the gradual introduction of 'payment by results' since 2003. NHS funding increases ran at record levels for five years until 2008/09, and had always been planned to be much slower after that. Now, however, despite a government commitment to increase the NHS budget in real terms until 2015, with growth at a mere 0.1 per cent it is under great pressure. Funding beyond 2015 may stall again, with further cuts already planned in overall public spending. The NHS therefore needs to secure the maximum gains from improved efficiency and productivity if it is to continue to meet rising demand.

Sources of funding

Taxation
Funding healthcare through taxation ensures universal access to services irrespective of ability to pay. About three-quarters of NHS funding in England comes from general taxation – the Consolidated Fund – and just under a fifth from the NHS element of national insurance.

The health service is the second biggest single item of public expenditure (after social security payments), and absorbs 18 per cent of money raised through tax and national insurance contributions (NICs).

General taxation is generally regarded as being a highly efficient way of financing healthcare: it means the Government has both a strong incentive and the capacity to control costs; administrative costs especially tend to be lower. As taxation draws revenue from a wide base, it helps minimise distortions in particular sectors of the economy. The social insurance element of NHS financing in the form of NICs paid by employees and employers, although relatively small, has been found to be highly progressive – that is, what people pay directly reflects what they can afford.

However, financing healthcare through taxation means the overall level of resources is constrained by what the Government judges the economy can afford and what is electorally viable, while choices between what services are and are not provided are made centrally. Many would argue that until 2000 the UK system went too far in controlling expenditure, leading to under-investment in the NHS compared with other countries over many years. The degree of individual choice available to patients has tended to be relatively limited, although current policy is trying to address this.

Charges
The NHS currently charges for a limited number of clinical services – in England mainly prescriptions, dental treatments, sight tests, glasses and contact lenses. These out-of-pocket payments account for about 2 per cent of NHS funding. The principle remains that they should be paid only by those who can afford them, so those who cannot are not discouraged from seeking advice and treatment. A wide range of exemptions applies, including in most cases young and elderly people and those who are unemployed or on low incomes.

Prescriptions, dental treatment, sight tests
Since April 2013, prescription charges in England have been £7.85 per item. NHS Wales abolished prescription charges in 2007 and NHS Scotland in 2011. Prescription charges in Northern Ireland were abolished in 2010, although it has considered reintroducing them. Complete abolition has been ruled out in England as it would reduce NHS revenue by about £450 million, but charges for cancer patients were ended in 2009. It is estimated that about 50 per cent of the population of England does not have to pay prescription charges. About 89 per cent of prescription items are dispensed free to patients.

Most courses of dental treatment cost £18 or £49, depending on their complexity. The maximum charge for complex dental treatment is £214. NHS dental charges raised £614 million in 2010/11. Sight test charges vary but are usually between £17 and £30, although they have been free in Scotland since 2006.

In addition, there are currently limited charges for non-clinical services such as single maternity rooms and car parking.

Recovering the costs of personal injury
Since the 1930s hospitals have been entitled by law to collect money for treating road traffic accident victims from drivers' insurance companies. Since 2007 the NHS has been able to recover costs from insurance companies for treating patients in all cases where personal injury compensation is paid. In 2011/12, the injury costs recovery scheme raised £183 million in England. The Compensation Recovery Unit, part of the

Department for Work and Pensions, collects the charges on the DH's behalf. They are:
- use of an NHS ambulance: £189
- flat rate for treatment without admission: £627
- daily rate for treatment with admission: £770
- maximum in any one case: £46,046.

Further information
Compensation Recovery Unit www.dwp.gov.uk/other-specialists/compensation-recovery-unit

Overseas visitors
Anyone who is lawfully 'ordinarily resident' in the UK is entitled to free NHS treatment in England, regardless of nationality. UK residents may be absent from the country for up to six months in a year before being considered for charges for NHS hospital treatment. British citizens who do not normally live in the UK may have to pay charges for NHS treatment, regardless of whether they have paid UK taxes and national insurance contributions, unless they are eligible for certain exemptions. British state pensioners who split their time between the UK and another European Economic Area member state are exempt from charges. Responsibility for deciding who is entitled to free treatment rests with the hospital providing the treatment.

Asylum seekers whose application for refuge in the UK is outstanding are entitled to use NHS services without charge, as are those refused asylum but unable to return home due to 'recognised barriers'. Unaccompanied children, including those in local authority care, are also exempt from charges. In any case, treatment in an A&E department or walk-in centre, family planning services, compulsory psychiatric treatment and treatment for certain communicable diseases are free to all.

Further information
Guidance on implementing the overseas visitors hospital charging regulations, DH, October 2012.

Resource allocation
The Treasury is responsible for overall public expenditure. It periodically conducts a spending review of all government departments, after which departments – including the DH – draw up structural reform plans, setting out what they expect to provide with their new resources.

Once the Treasury makes its allocation to the DH, the Secretary of State decides how it is divided between the NHS and public health, making grants to local authorities for their public health responsibilities. In 2013/14, the Secretary of State has allocated £95 billion to NHS England for the NHS and £2.7 billion for public health.

Resources for the NHS are passed to NHS England, which then decides:
• how much it will spend commissioning primary care
• how much it will spend commissioning specialised services
• how much to allocate to CCGs for them to commission secondary and community services.

NHS England calculates practice-level budgets and allocates these directly to CCGs, which are responsible for managing the combined commissioning budgets of their member practices. Allocations are made according to a formula devised by the Advisory Committee on Resource Allocation (ACRA), which takes into account NHS England's duty to reduce inequalities in access to services and in patient outcomes.

Currently NHS England has concerns that the formula, if used on its own to redistribute funding, would result in higher growth for areas that already have the best health outcomes compared to those with the worst. It is therefore conducting a fundamental review of the approach to allocations, drawing on ACRA's expert advice and involving others whose functions impact on outcomes and inequalities. It is intended to be completed in time to inform 2014/15 allocations.

Capital

Capital investment is expenditure – typically on buildings or large items of equipment – that will continue to provide benefits into the future. To count as NHS capital, spending must generally be on assets that individually cost £5,000 or more and are recorded on the balance sheet as fixed assets.

The NHS's main sources of capital are government funds, receipts from land sales and the private finance initiative. NHS England sets capital limits for each clinical commissioning group.

Foundation trusts are free to reinvest all cash generated from their activities to maintain and replace their assets. They may also borrow capital under 'prudential borrowing' arrangements if their projections of

Spotlight on policy: **payment by results**

In a far-reaching change to the way money flows through the NHS in England between commissioners and providers, a system of payment by results has been gradually introduced. The aim is to ensure funding follows the patient, to underpin policy on increasing patient choice among a variety of providers.

The intention is to provide a transparent system for paying providers, which encourages activity and so helps keep waiting times short. Commissioners purchase the volume of activity they require for their populations, but instead of drawing up block agreements as previously, providers are paid for the activity they undertake. A tariff derived from national reference costs removed prices from local negotiation, so that commissioners focus instead on gains in patient choice, quality, shorter waiting time, volumes of activity and efficiency.

Payment by results began in a limited way in 2003/04, and has been gradually extended: it now covers about 60 per cent of acute hospital income and a third of CCG budgets. Each year, changes to the tariff are 'sense-checked' for anomalies that could lead to perverse incentives and 'road-tested' before their introduction to enable the service to get used to the new tariff.

A code of conduct for payment by results sets out core principles, ground rules for organisational behaviour and expectations of how the system should operate – and is intended to minimise disputes. Responsibility for setting all pricing will rest jointly with NHS England and Monitor from January 2014.

In 2010/11 'best practice tariffs' to provide incentives and reimburse the costs of high-quality care were introduced for four high-volume areas with significant unexplained variation in practice. After evaluation it was decided to introduce more best practice tariffs for 2013/14.

For 2013/14, tariff prices have been reduced by 1.1 per cent, with pricing in general reduced by 1.3 per cent – a 4 per cent efficiency requirement offsetting pay and price inflation of 2.7 per cent.

Further information
Payment by results guidance for 2013–14, DH, February 2013.
Code of conduct for payment by results in 2013–14, DH, February 2013.
A simple guide to payment by results, DH, November 2012.
Best practice tariffs and their impact, Audit Commission, November 2012.
*A qualitative and quantitative evaluation of the introduction of best practice tariffs:
an evaluation report commissioned by the Department of Health*, Universities of
Nottingham and Manchester, October 2012.

future cash flows show they would be able to afford to pay back the
sum with interest. Monitor assigns each foundation trust a 'prudential
borrowing limit', fixing the amount of debt it may take on.

Private finance initiative (PFI)

PFI involves a public–private partnership between an NHS organisation
and a private sector consortium that makes private capital available for
health service projects.

The private sector consortium will usually include a construction
company, a funding organisation and a facilities management provider.
Contracts for major PFI schemes may be for 30 years or more and are
typically DBFO (design, build, finance and operate) projects. This means
the private sector partner is responsible for:
• designing the facilities (based on the requirements specified by the NHS)
• building the facilities (to time and at a fixed cost)
• financing the capital cost (with the return to be recovered through
  continuing to make the facilities available and meeting NHS
  requirements)
• operating the facilities (providing facilities management and other
  support services).

One aim of PFI is to reduce the overall risks associated with procuring
new assets and services for the NHS, as well as to improve the quality
and cost-effectiveness of public services. But it has sparked considerable
debate. Critics question whether PFI really provides long-term value for
money for the NHS, and claim services have been cut in some cases to
make schemes affordable.

By 2010, there were 103 PFI schemes in place across England. Annual payment costs were over £1.2 billion in 2011/12, and are expected to rise to £2.3 billion a year by 2030. Attempts are being made to reduce these costs, with 'hit squads' examining PFI contracts to identify savings. But the likelihood of PFI contracts being renegotiated in favour of NHS providers is limited, particularly given that the contracts are underwritten by the Treasury and so investors have little incentive to make concessions in recouping their investment. Recently, the Treasury proposed a new finance scheme to replace PFI, called PF2, which is designed to be more transparent and would see the public sector act as a minority shareholder in future projects.

NHS Local Improvement Finance Trust (LIFT)
NHS LIFT aims to encourage investment in primary care and community-based facilities with the aim of refurbishing or replacing them. It is similar to PFI, except that it is a joint venture between the NHS, the private sector partner, local authorities and GPs.

Community Health Partnerships (CHP), a public–private partnership between the DH and Partnerships UK, was set up to invest money in NHS LIFT and help attract additional private funding; the DH became the sole owner in 2006. At local level, NHS LIFT is not a single trust but a series of local public–private partnerships between the NHS, the private sector, CHP and local authorities. The resulting partnership is a LIFT company, which is a local joint venture.

More than 300 new community facilities have opened in the last ten years as part of the LIFT programme, and 49 local LIFT schemes are renting accommodation to GPs, pharmacists, opticians, dentists and others on a lease basis. Schemes may now include clinical and facilities management services as well as buildings and maintenance. The total value of the LIFT programme is over £2.5 billion.

The DH also wholly owns NHS Property Services Ltd (or PropCo), a sister company to CHP set up to maintain, manage and develop a large part of the NHS estate worth about £5 billion and comprising 3,600 facilities. It employs 3,000 staff.

Further information
CHP **www.communityhealthpartnerships.co.uk**
NHS Property Services **www.property.nhs.uk**

NHS spending

Tough times

The NHS faces an unprecedented financial dilemma: the supply of funding is struggling to match the growing rate of demand for healthcare. This is caused by rising costs within the NHS, driven by:

• increased demand
• innovation
• lifestyle choices
• mental health and social care needs.

In the NHS Confederation's 2013 survey of NHS leaders, 62 per cent described the current financial position as 'the worst they had ever experienced' or 'very serious', and 83 per cent expected financial pressures to increase in the year ahead.

The Government's first comprehensive spending review, covering 2011–15, promised that NHS average annual real-terms funding would increase by 0.1 per cent – despite planned annual spending cuts of 2.9 per cent in real terms across the rest of the public sector.

NHS funding (£ billion) – England

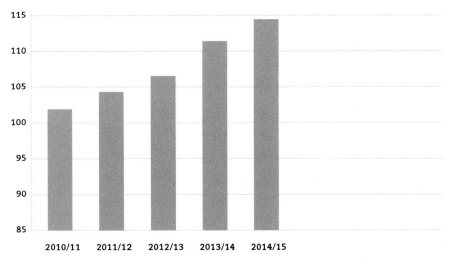

Source: HM Treasury

When inflation is factored in, the reality of the situation facing the NHS hits home. Health inflation has traditionally run ahead of headline inflation, mainly because of ever-increasing demand from patients and the cost of technology. Using inflation figures published alongside the 2013 Budget, NHS funding declined in real terms in 2010/11 before increasing slightly in 2011/12 and 2012/13. This real-terms freeze 'represents the tightest period of funding in the last 50 years of the NHS', according to the Nuffield Trust and the Institute for Fiscal Studies. In recent years, DH 'underspends' have been transferred to other departments (see opposite); if this trend continues, spending growth is likely to decline further.

NHS real-terms expenditure (£ billion) – England

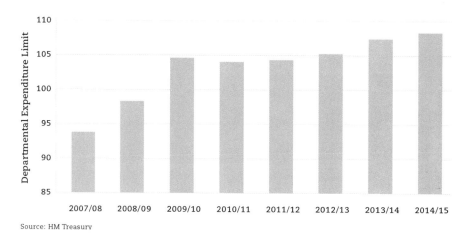

Source: HM Treasury

Overall financial balance

The NHS has secured much more effective control over its finances in recent years, with healthy overall surpluses achieved in each of the past seven years. Yet 34 organisations (around 8 per cent) still reported a deficit totalling £356 million in their annual accounts for 2011/12.

One way of achieving such healthy surpluses was for primary care trusts' budgets to be 'top-sliced'. Since 2010, this has amounted to 2 per cent of the budgets, with some of it released for specific non-recurrent proposals.

This looks set to continue under the new commissioning arrangements. While in theory the NHS was meant to be able to access the surplus funds in the years ahead, £2.9 billion of underspend in 2010/11 and 2011/12 has been returned to the Treasury, with only £316 million of the latter year's surplus carried over to 2012/13 to be spent on health services. In 2012/13 the NHS underspent its revenue budget by £1.4 billion and its capital budget by £800 million.

Efficiency

The consultancy company McKinsey suggested in 2009 that the NHS should make up to £20 billion of efficiency savings by 2015. This is now being implemented under the QIPP programme (Quality, Innovation, Productivity and Prevention), also known as the 'Nicholson challenge' after NHS England's chief executive. He has suggested that QIPP savings can be delivered from:

- administration and management (£8 billion)
- tariff payments (£8 billion)
- service redesign (£4 billion).

The NHS achieved savings of £5.8 billion in 2011/12, including £1.9 billion in the final quarter of the year alone. The National Audit Office noted this figure was close to the forecast of £5.9 billion, but warned of 'limited assurance that all the reported savings were achieved' and expressed concern about the NHS's ability 'to generate new efficiency savings in future years'.

Future funding

The 2013 Budget confirmed that NHS funding would be protected until 2016. Debate about future funding has been growing, particularly regarding whether the NHS budget will continue to be protected when further real-terms public spending cuts are planned up to at least 2017/18.

The Nuffield Trust has estimated the NHS in England will have up to £34 billion of additional financial pressure to cope with by 2021/22 if the budget is frozen in real terms. This is the case even if the £20 billion of QIPP savings to 2015 are achieved in full, and would require continued annual 4 per cent efficiency savings. If the budget was to rise in line with national income projections, then the gap would still be up to £14 billion, with efficiency savings of 2 per cent needed to meet the gap.

Further information

Tough times, tough choices: being open and honest about NHS finance, NHS Confederation, March 2013.

Briefing 259: Tough times, tough choices – being open and honest about NHS finance, NHS Confederation, March 2013.

Factsheet: Tough times, tough choices – an overview of NHS finances, NHS Confederation, March 2013.

Factsheet: Tough times, tough choices – how does the NHS financial situation compare? NHS Confederation, March 2013.

Where the money goes (2011/12) – £ billion

% increase since the previous year shown in brackets

1 General and acute care: £40.204 (3.2%)

2 Primary healthcare: £21.637 (1.2%)

3 Community services: £9.119 (8.4%)

4 Mental illness: £8.608 (2.8%)

5 Other secondary care: £3.170 (5.1%)

6 Maternity: £2.621 (3.5%)

7 A&E: £2.326 (4.6%)

8 Learning difficulties: £1.416 (45.2% decrease*)

*Result of some functions being transferred to local authorities.

Source: The Audit Commission

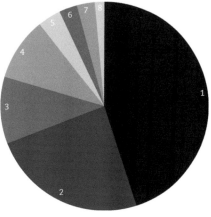

NHS Shared Business Services

NHS Shared Business Services was launched as a joint venture between the DH and a private sector company in 2005, building on an earlier shared financial services initiative. SBS provides finance and accounting, payroll, human resources and procurement services so that frontline organisations can concentrate on patient care. With 1,200 employees at 13 locations in England and 550 staff in India, it processes £43 billion worth of payments a year.
www.sbs.nhs.uk

NHS Business Services Authority

This special health authority was set up in 2006 to be the main processing facility for payment, reimbursement, remuneration and reconciliation for NHS patients, employees and others. For example, it manages the NHS pension scheme, reimburses dentists and pharmacists, and administers the European health insurance card in the UK. It was formed from the Dental Practice Board, NHS Pensions Agency and the Prescription Pricing Authority.
www.nhsbsa.nhs.uk

NHS Supply Chain

NHS Supply Chain is a single organisation that provides procurement, logistics, e-commerce and customer and supplier support. Its 2,400 staff buy and deliver over 620,000 products for more than 1,000 healthcare organisations. It aims to save £1.2 billion for the NHS, and is operated by DHL under a ten-year contract with the NHS Business Services Authority.
www.supplychain.nhs.uk

NHS Protect

NHS Protect leads work to protect NHS staff and resources from crime. It has national responsibility for tackling fraud, violence, bribery, corruption, criminal damage, theft and other unlawful action such as market-fixing. It also leads work on NHS emergency and counter-terrorism preparedness, national data analysis and risk assessment, anti-fraud and pro-security research. In addition, it provides NHS anti-fraud services to the Welsh Government.
www.nhsbsa.nhs.uk/Protect

07 Staffing and human resources

As the UK's largest employer – indeed, one of the largest employers in the world – the NHS attaches special importance to good human resources policy and practice. Staff costs account for about 75 per cent of hospital spending. Effective recruitment, retention and remuneration of a well-trained and well-motivated workforce are seen as crucial factors in achieving ambitions for patient care.

The era of funding growth during the first decade of this century saw significant expansion in the NHS workforce and revised contracts to reflect changing patterns of care. The NHS currently has over 1.3 million staff in more than 300 different roles. Improving staff productivity and efficiency as spending diminishes is now a key theme. Organisations must also do their utmost to engage staff in designing ways of improving services, as well as fostering leadership at all levels. NHS commitments to staff, and staff's responsibilities, form a major part of the NHS Constitution (see page 131).

Further information
Liberating the NHS: developing the healthcare workforce – from design to delivery, DH, January 2012.

Workforce planning

The Department of Health now has much less direct involvement in planning and developing the healthcare workforce, in line with the Government's policy of devolving responsibility for decision-making as close to the front line as possible. A new national body, Health Education England, now provides national leadership for planning and developing the whole healthcare and public health workforce, while local education and training boards (LETBs) articulate local needs. The Government expects to see healthcare providers with local clinical leadership take a lead role in planning and developing their workforce.

Health Education England
HEE oversees workforce planning, education and training, as well as supporting local arrangements for planning and commissioning education and training. It took over the functions of Medical Education England (which covered medicine, dentistry, pharmacy and healthcare science), the allied health professional advisory board and the nursing and midwifery professional advisory board.

HEE's purpose is to ensure the health workforce has the right skills and is available in the right numbers. Key functions are:

- providing national leadership on planning and developing the workforce
- authorising and supporting development of LETBs
- promoting education and training responsive to changing needs, including responsibility for recruiting medical trainees
- allocating and accounting for NHS education and training resources and the outcomes achieved
- ensuring the supply of the professionally qualified clinical workforce
- assisting the spread of innovation across the NHS
- achieving the aims of the National Education Outcomes Framework.

HEE's main focus is on professionally qualified staff whose education and training is funded through the multi-professional education and training budget, almost £5 billion a year. It is playing a key role in the proposed changes to nurse training. HEE is accountable to the Secretary of State, and has about 150 staff, many in LETBs.

Further information
Introducing Health Education England: our strategic intent, HEE, February 2013.
http://hee.nhs.uk

Local education and training boards
The 13 LETBs enable NHS employers, education providers and health professionals to work together to plan and commission education and training. They have flexibility to support local priorities in innovation and workforce development. LETBs are statutory committees of HEE. Their functions include:

- developing a skills and development strategy for the local health workforce
- collecting local workforce data and plans
- accounting for education and training funding allocated by HEE
- securing the quality of education and training programmes
- supporting access to continuing professional development
- working in partnership with universities, clinical academics, other education providers and those investing in research and innovation
- working with local authorities and health and wellbeing boards
- working with HEE to develop national strategy and priorities.

LETBs determine their own investment plans and take responsibility for the education and training they decide to commission, subject to following HEE's national strategic direction.

Centre for Workforce Intelligence

The Centre for Workforce Intelligence (CfWI), which reports to HEE, has three key functions:

- helping senior leaders drive workforce planning, strengthening the influence of workforce planners and connecting different parts of the system
- providing workforce intelligence to the health and social care system to inform decisions
- providing the support, resources and best practice to improve the effectiveness of workforce planning at local, regional and national levels.

www.cfwi.org.uk

Number of staff (000s)

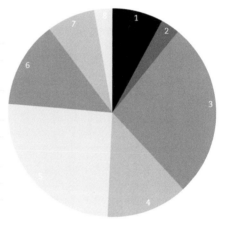

1 Hospital and community medical and dental staff: 106

2 GPs: 40

3 Qualified nursing, midwifery and health visiting staff: 370

4 Other qualified scientific, therapeutic and technical staff: 171

5 Support to clinical staff: 347

6 Hospital and community central functions and estates: 182

7 GP practice staff: 101

8 Managers and senior managers: 38

Source: NHS Workforce Census Bulletin, 2001–2011, Health and Social Care Information Centre.

Social Partnership Forum

The NHS Social Partnership Forum, set up in 1998 and revised in 2007 and 2012, brings together NHS trade unions, NHS Employers, the DH, NHS England and HEE to discuss current issues and develop joint initiatives to tackle national problems. It meets five times a year, three times as a wider group and twice as a smaller steering group, and is chaired by a health minister.

Current work priorities are:

- supporting staff through change and transfer
- workforce implications of QIPP (see page 119)
- staff morale and engagement
- strengthening partnership
- responding to emerging issues.

NHS Employers
NHS Employers represents employing organisations in the health service in
England on workforce issues. It reflects employers' views and acts on their
behalf in four priority areas:
• pay and negotiations
• recruitment and planning the workforce
• healthy and productive workplaces
• employment policy and practice.

NHS Employers, set up in 2004, is part of the NHS Confederation. The DH
sets the broad framework within which it operates, but employers
themselves drive the agenda. Its policy board oversees the strategic
direction and governance of the organisation, with members drawn from
across the NHS.
www.nhsemployers.org

The Forum has produced the NHS Staff Passport toolkit, a guide for staff
facing transfer that includes information on employment standards and
rights they can expect when transferring from a job either within the NHS,
or from a job within the NHS to another organisation.

Further information
Partnership agreement: an agreement between DH, NHS Employers and NHS trade unions,
Social Partnership Forum/DH, February 2012.
www.socialpartnershipforum.org

NHS Careers
NHS Careers is a service providing information on careers in the NHS in
England. It consists of a telephone and email helpline, website, literature
and supporting services for NHS employers, schools, colleges and careers
advisers. Launched in 1999, it aims to raise awareness among the potential
future workforce of the 350 careers the NHS offers. It has developed a
service for 14–19-year-olds to find out what working in the NHS is like,
and another where undergraduates on clinical and non-clinical courses
in England can look at their options for a career in the NHS.
www.nhscareers.nhs.uk
www.stepintothenhs.nhs.uk
www.whatcanidowithmydegree.nhs.uk

NHS Jobs

NHS Jobs is an online recruitment service offering details of job vacancies throughout the NHS in England and Wales. Launched in 2003, it provides employers with online tools to manage every stage of the recruitment cycle. Each month it carries details of around 20,000 career opportunities in the NHS, attracts 6 million visits and receives job applications from more than 250,000 jobseekers. Ninety per cent of NHS job applications are made through the website. Every NHS organisation in England and Wales is registered to advertise with NHS Jobs, which is estimated to have saved the NHS over £240 million in advertising and recruitment administration costs since its launch.
www.jobs.nhs.uk

Pay and pensions

Pay accounts for about 40 per cent of NHS spending, and 65 to 70 per cent in acute and mental health trusts. The pay and conditions of NHS staff are developed mainly through collective bargaining between the NHS and staff organisations, which also represent staff on a wide range of other employment issues. Most staff are members of trade unions or professional associations, and the NHS seeks 'partnership working' on key employment issues. Most NHS staff organisations have a professional and collective bargaining role. NHS Employers negotiates conditions of service and national contracts with the unions on behalf of employers through the NHS Staff Council, and represents employers' views in the pay review process. GPs are independent self-employed contractors, and the general medical services contract (see opposite) is negotiated by the British Medical Association and NHS Employers.

Agenda for Change

Agenda for Change was the most significant reform of NHS pay since the creation of the health service in 1948. It applies to 1.3 million NHS staff across the UK, with the exception of doctors, dentists and the most senior managers.

The system is underpinned by a job evaluation scheme specifically designed for the NHS and by the NHS knowledge and skills framework, which supports personal development and career progression.

Agenda for Change was designed to:
• deliver fair pay for non-medical staff based on the principle of equal pay for work of equal value

- provide better links between pay and career progression through the NHS knowledge and skills framework
- harmonise terms and conditions of service such as annual leave, hours and sick pay, and more recently for work performed in unsocial hours.

Staff are placed in one of nine pay bands on the basis of their knowledge, responsibility, skills and effort needed for the job rather than on the basis of their job title.

The terms and conditions of service for all staff directly employed by NHS organisations under Agenda for Change are set out in the NHS Staff Council's NHS terms and conditions of service handbook.

All NHS staff earning more than £21,000 had their pay frozen for two years in April 2011. Rises from April 2013 have been capped at 1 per cent.

Further information
NHS terms and conditions of service handbook, NHS Staff Council, NHS Staff Council, March 2013.
The NHS knowledge and skills framework: essential guide for NHS boards, NHS Employers, 2007.
The NHS knowledge and skills framework (KSF): essential guide for NHS staff, NHS Employers, 2007.

Contract for GPs
A new GP contract for general medical services (GMS) was implemented across the UK in 2004, with annual revisions made after negotiations between NHS Employers and the British Medical Association's General Practitioners Committee (GPC). The contract aims to reward practices for providing high-quality care, improve GPs' working lives and ensure patients benefit from a wider range of services in the community.

The GMS contract is between the practice and NHS England rather than with each GP. This is intended to give practices greater freedom to design services for local needs while encouraging better teamworking and skill-mix.

A key component of the GMS contract is the Quality and Outcomes Framework (QOF) which resources and rewards practices for delivering high-quality care (see page 76). QOF payments increasingly reflect the prevalence of long-term health conditions, to help address health inequalities by ensuring proportionately greater funding for practices in deprived areas.

Contracts for other doctors and dentists

The current consultants' contract, introduced in 2003, is designed to provide a more effective system of planning and timetabling consultants' duties and activities for the NHS. It gives NHS employers the ability to manage consultants' time in ways that best meet local service needs and priorities. For consultants, it means greater transparency about the commitments expected of them and greater clarity over the support they need from employers to make the maximum effective contribution to improving patient services.

The current contractual arrangements for doctors in hospital and public health training have been in force since December 2000. Junior doctors' hours have been reduced to levels set in the European working-time directive: a maximum of 48 hours per week averaged over 26 weeks.

A new contract for staff grade and associate specialist doctors was agreed in 2008. It applies to 13,000 non-consultant career grade NHS doctors and to all entrants to the new specialty doctor grade. Annual appraisal, job planning and objective setting are essential components of the new contract.

A salaried dentists' contract was implemented in early 2008. A new single pay spine covers dentists, senior dentists, specialist dentists and managerial dentists. The new pay structure is supported by mandatory annual appraisals and job planning to assist career development.

A new community pharmacy contract was implemented in England in 2005, allowing pharmacies to offer an expanded range of clinical services.

Pensions, retirement and redundancy

All NHS staff automatically become members of the NHS pension scheme, but they can choose not to join or leave at any time. The scheme for England and Wales underwent significant changes in 2008. Clear processes and procedures for handling absence and supporting staff through rehabilitation, redeployment or ill health retirements were part of this. About 30,000 staff retire from the NHS every year.

The Government proposed changes to all public service pension schemes, as recommended by the Independent Public Service Pensions Commission led by Lord Hutton, in order to make them sustainable and to save £2.8 billion by 2014/15. Increases in employee contributions are being phased in over three years from April 2012. Other revisions to the pension scheme itself will be implemented from April 2015.

Redundancy arrangements for all staff directly employed by NHS organisations, except very senior managers and staff covered by the Doctors' and Dentists' Review Body, are included in the *NHS terms and conditions of service handbook*.

Further information
NHS pension scheme: consultation on the NHS pension scheme, additional voluntary contributions, and injury benefits (amendment) regulations 2013 – Government response, DH, March 2013.
NHS Pension Scheme **www.nhsbsa.nhs.uk/pensions**

The NHS as an employer

The NHS recognises staff as its greatest asset and knows that to recruit and retain the right people it needs to practise excellence in employment. This includes treating staff with respect and supporting them in their work; valuing equality and diversity; ensuring a healthy workplace; offering flexible working; and providing training and opportunities for development.

Staff 'engagement' is a high priority for the NHS as it can improve morale, productivity, organisational performance and patient experience. Research indicates that staff satisfaction – and retention, discretionary effort and productivity – are closely associated with how staff feel about their employer and their sense of engagement with their workplace. The degree of staff involvement in planning and delivering services is an important factor in this, while increasing evidence shows direct links between staff satisfaction and the patient experience.

After being updated in 2013, the NHS Constitution makes seven pledges to staff:
• to provide a positive working environment and promote supportive, open cultures
• to provide all staff with clear roles and responsibilities and rewarding jobs for teams and individuals
• to provide all staff with personal development, access to appropriate training and the support of line management to enable them to fulfil their potential
• to provide support and opportunities for staff to maintain their health, wellbeing and safety
• to engage staff in decisions that affect them and the services they provide individually, through representative organisations and local partnership working arrangements. All staff will be empowered to put forward better ways to deliver better and safer services

- to have a process for staff to raise an internal grievance
- to encourage and support all staff in raising concerns at the earliest reasonable opportunity about safety, malpractice and wrongdoing at work, responding to and investigating concerns.

The Constitution places six legal duties on staff and 12 expectations. Key ones stipulate that staff should:
- accept professional accountability and maintain the standards of professional practice
- not discriminate against patients or staff and adhere to equal opportunities, equality and human rights legislation
- protect the confidentiality of personal information they hold.

The Government is consulting on further changes that would include a responsibility for staff to treat patients with compassion, dignity and respect, and a statutory 'duty of candour' that means staff must be open and honest with patients about mistakes.

The tenth national NHS staff survey took place from September to December 2012, and asked 203,000 staff about their experiences, with 50 per cent responding. Sixty-three per cent of NHS staff said that if a friend or relative needed treatment they would be happy with the standard of care provided by their organisation. The proportion of staff receiving appraisals improved to 83 per cent, but only 36 per cent said these were well structured. Only 40 per cent were satisfied that their organisation valued their work, but the proportion indicating they would recommend their organisation as a place to work has increased from 51 to 55 per cent. Only 35 per cent said communication between senior managers and staff was effective, and less than a third reported that senior managers acted on feedback from staff. Despite this, 74 per cent said they were able to make suggestions on how they could improve the work of their team or department. The overall index of staff engagement showed a small increase.

Further information
The NHS Constitution for England, March 2013.
National NHS Staff Survey Coordination Centre **www.nhsstaffsurveys.com**

Appendix

The structure of the NHS in Scotland[1]

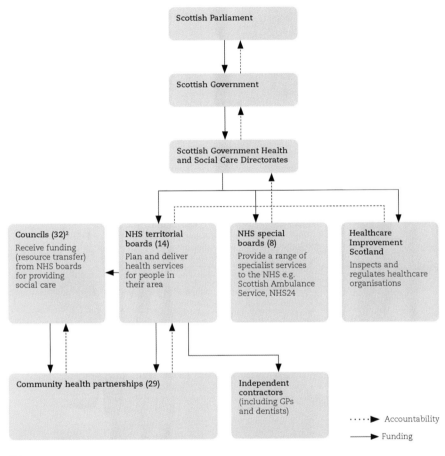

Notes

1. The Scottish Government has announced plans to integrate adult health and social care services.
2. The main source of funding for councils is the Scottish Government Communities and Local Government Directorates.

Source: Audit Scotland

The structure of the NHS in Wales

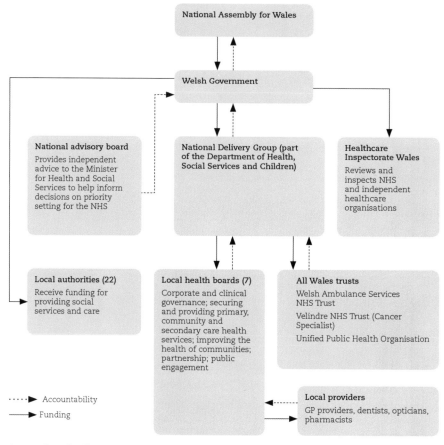

National Assembly for Wales

Welsh Government

National advisory board

Provides independent advice to the Minister for Health and Social Services to help inform decisions on priority setting for the NHS

National Delivery Group (part of the Department of Health, Social Services and Children)

Healthcare Inspectorate Wales

Reviews and inspects NHS and independent healthcare organisations

Local authorities (22)

Receive funding for providing social services and care

Local health boards (7)

Corporate and clinical governance; securing and providing primary, community and secondary care health services; improving the health of communities; partnership; public engagement

All Wales trusts

Welsh Ambulance Services NHS Trust

Velindre NHS Trust (Cancer Specialist)

Unified Public Health Organisation

Local providers

GP providers, dentists, opticians, pharmacists

· · · ·▶ Accountability

———▶ Funding

Source: Wales Audit Office

The structure of the NHS in Northern Ireland

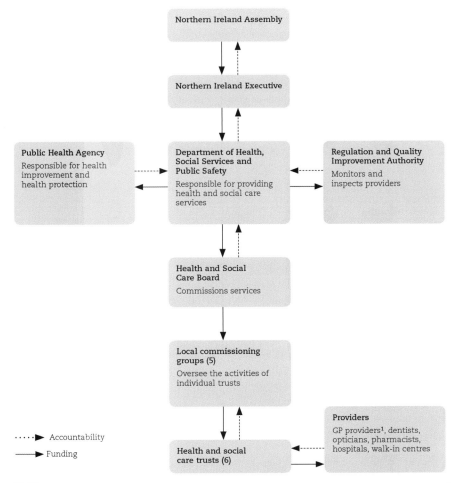

Notes

1. GPs in Northern Ireland are contracted directly by the Health and Social Care Board and so they receive funding from, and are directly accountable to, the Board rather then the health and social care trusts.

Source: Northern Ireland Audit Office

Acknowledgements

The NHS Confederation is grateful to all those involved in the production of this edition of *The concise NHS handbook* (formerly known as *The NHS handbook* and before 2008 as *The pocket guide*). Particular thanks are due to:

- our sponsor, NHS Professionals
- those organisations that have kindly allowed us to reproduce diagrams and other materials
- Grade Design, for designing and typesetting this year's handbook and also for designing the front cover
- Peter Mac for the cover illustration
- Caroline Ball for her expert editing and proofreading.

We are also grateful to our members and other customers who have provided valuable feedback on previous editions of the handbook/pocket guide, to enable us to make year-on-year improvements.

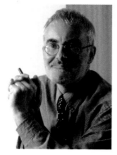

The author

Peter Davies is a freelance writer and editor. He has written extensively on health policy and management issues, for which he won a major award from the Medical Journalists Association. He was editor of *Health Service Journal* from 1993 to 2002, and has contributed a regular column to *Guardian Unlimited*. He is married with two children and lives in London.